Race For Sobriety

Rochelle Moncourtois-Baxter

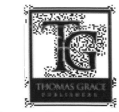

Thomas Grace Publishers

Acknowledgements

Thank you to my husband for always being there for me no matter what. You are my rock and sobriety brought us even closer together. I have the utmost respect and love for you. I could not have made it through this journey without your support. I am grateful for you and our twin girls. Thank you to Kim. You are my mentor, role model, and motivator. My journey to becoming sober and an Ironman triathlete would not have been possible without your love and support. You are an amazing woman and I will always look up to you.

Dedication

I would like to dedicate this book to my parents, Paul and Alyce Moncourtois. They have always been there for me through the thick and thin. I couldn't have made my dreams possible without them.

Table of Contents

Introduction
What is Alcoholism?

There is absolutely nothing that can prepare someone for the struggles and misery that alcoholism will bring. It is a disease that will slowly creep up on you and quickly destroy your life. It waits and hibernates until the right moment comes along. It doesn't care about background, skin color, socioeconomics, physical appearance, gender, or age. It can be present in any type of individual.

There are numerous arguments about whether or not alcoholism is an illness. From my own personal experience, I believe there is something in an alcoholic's brain that is definitely different from what would be considered a "normal" brain. When an alcoholic picks up a drink, their brain overrides all common sense thinking and they are unable to stop drinking once they start. One drink isn't enough nor is a thousand. This illness isn't something that can be controlled without intervention of some kind.

There is no magic pill to get rid of what alcoholics call "the craving," which is that uncontrollable urge to consume alcohol. It is unlike anything else I have experienced in my lifetime. In the Big Book of Alcoholics Anonymous, it is referred to as a "phenomenon" and is powerful and can totally take over and cause an alcoholic to lose all control. When an alcoholic takes even the tiniest sip of alcohol, it immediately warms, numbs, and leaves a feeling of satisfaction. Unfortunately, this feeling of satisfaction is false and temporary and the continued consumption will only make things worse.

An alcoholic's "drunk" is very different from that which a non-alcoholic or "normie" would experience. An alcoholic's drunk causes many problems and chaos every single time a drink is consumed and the ensuing morning-after hangover is so awful that more alcohol is consumed in an effort to get rid of the hangover. This, in reality, is just another excuse an alcoholic uses to start the cycle all over again. None of this behavior is exhibited by a normie. Yes, a normie can drink to excess and experience the pain and suffering of a hangover, but drinking the morning-after doesn't occur.

All of this may sound like pure insanity but that is just what this illness does to a person. One definition of insanity is repeating the same thing over and over and expecting the same results. The insanity in alcoholics takes many forms such as self- pity, being a master manipulator and liar, blaming others for their problems, or losing all control. Like the definition says, these things are repeated, the same results occur, but no lesson is learned and thus the cycle starts all over again.

The reasons people start drinking vary and can range from growing up in an unhealthy environment to having no issues at all. Alcoholism is an illness that stays dormant, emerges when least expected, and becomes apparent when life reaches the unmanageability stage. There are many red flags that can indicate that alcohol use is interfering with everyday life. Losing one job after another because of hangover issues or missing important family events are just two examples. Alcoholism can destroy every aspect of someone's life including relationships with family and friends, career loss, and financial ruin.

There are many different types of alcoholics. I was considered a binge drinker. A binge drinker doesn't drink 24/7 but when they do, it's two to three days of non-stop drinking. Some binge drinkers can be what are considered blackout drinkers who drink until they cannot remember anything that occurred during their drinking binge. Every type of alcoholic drinker is dangerous whether a daily drinker or a once-a-month drinker.

The illness slowly creeps up on an individual and the amount of alcohol consumed or the type of drinker doesn't make a difference. I refer to alcoholism and addiction as "little demons." These demons set out to destroy a life and can even cause death unless help is sought. If the desire is there to change the behaviors and the environments that are contributing to the addiction, then it is possible to overcome.

Until that happens, one excuse after another will impede forward progress toward recovery. That is how I lived my life for six years. I found any excuse to pick up a bottle of alcohol and drink. Then I denied that I had the illness and made more excuses to continue with my life of drinking. I had to reach the very low point in my life, admit I was an alcoholic, want to make the necessary changes, and seek professional help in order to beat those demons. That was 6 years ago and I never once looked back on my life of addiction.

Chapter 1
Growing Up Alcoholic

Some alcoholics say that they grew up in an unstable and unhealthy environment that contributed to their drinking career. Others say they grew up in what is considered a normal, functional household. I am one of those alcoholics. I grew up in a household that was warm, loving, healthy and very stable. I was fortunate to have a dad, mom, and a younger brother always by my side.

Families can play a very significant role in an alcoholic's upbringing and how they deal with life in general. Both my parents were not alcoholics or addicts. They were considered normies, a name for a nonalcoholic, and never had problems with alcohol. As I mentioned in the Introduction alcoholism is believed to be genetic. I can't say whether or not that is true in my case because no one on either side of my family had real serious dependency issues. I truly believe that somehow I got that one gene that led to it. People may argue whether or not alcohol and drug issues are all the fault of the parent. I can say that in my case it had nothing to do with my family background and how I was raised. My alcoholism is something I was born with but it didn't become an issue until I was older.

This is why I chose this chapter's title, "Growing Up Alcoholic." I believe my alcoholism wasn't a reflection on my childhood. It became something which caused me great grief later in life. I will elaborate on this in subsequent chapters. All I know is I grew up in a household that some children can only dream about and I'm forever grateful for that. My relations with each person in my immediate family were very significant during my drinking years. Everything I'm about to tell you is what led up to my out of control drinking, my recovery, and my journey to becoming an Ironman.

My mother has always been a very busy go-getter, and an all-around beautiful type of person. She grew up as someone who wanted to work hard to get where she wanted in life. She was a full time businesswoman and fitness instructor. I was born when my mother was twenty eight, two years after she married my dad. She was already well into her career and very financially stable. As a young girl, this is the type of woman I wanted to be, the real go-getter. I think having a mother that I looked up to was very significant because she was a good role model growing up.

My mother wanted the best for me and helped me throughout my childhood. My relationship with her as a child was a very normal mother/daughter relationship. When I was hurt or felt sick, I went to my mother like most children do. I sought comfort from her when I had childhood problems. One time as she was curling my hair for a professional photography shoot, she accidentally burned my neck with the curling iron. As I began crying hysterically, she comforted me and apologized for the pain she had inflicted. This is just one of the many examples that show how what a normal relationship we had. She was always there for me and provided advice and comfort. It is my belief that a mother should always be there for her children and my mother was that for me. She wanted me to succeed in life and started teaching me great life lessons from an early age.

You know the saying, "like mother, like daughter?" Well, my mother lived and breathed fitness just as I do now. I feel as though I was destined to be involved in fitness one way or another since her water broke while pregnant with me teaching an aerobics class. I was surrounded by fitness because of her healthy lifestyle. As a child I sometimes emulated her by putting on fitness gear and teaching a pretend class. I looked up to her because everything she did was so positive and seemed to make her happy.

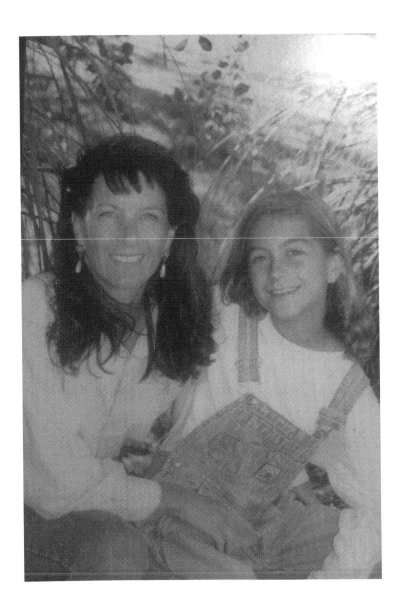

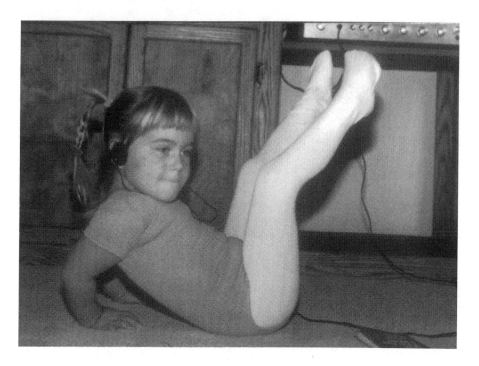

I even adopted her healthy eating habits as a young child, which carried through to adulthood. As a child you tend to "copy" what your parents do, including what they eat and whether they exercise. I closely observed her healthy choices in life. As a child I wanted to look just like her when I grew up. I knew I would always be involved with fitness and healthy eating because of the lifestyle she role-modeled. She was the greatest mom I could have asked for.

My father has always been a very loving, caring, smart, and handsome man. I had the type of relationship with him that most girls dream about. My father was always there for me. He went out of his way to make me happy and made my childhood wonderful. He was one of those men who would paint my toenails and then paint his just to make me smile and be happy.

I looked up to my father in a way that gave us a close relationship. When I looked at him I knew I wanted to marry someone just like him. He taught me how a gentleman should treat a woman and how a lady should act. I am one of those women who can say my father is my hero and will always be the first man in my life.

An early childhood memory is one I look upon with great fondness. I was at a swimming pool and other kids were daring each other to dive off the high diving board. My father looked at me and told me that I was brave enough to go show them how it is done. At just five years old I wanted to make him proud. I walked right up to the high school kids and told them I was going to show them how it is done and then jumped right in! I looked over at my father and he had a big smile on his face. I knew that one little act of bravery made him a proud father. That moment of making him proud was one I wanted to continue for the rest of my life.

I believe that a healthy relationship between a father and a daughter is extremely important and I was fortunate enough to have that with my father. I am what they call a "daddy's girl." When I really wanted something I would smile and stick out my tongue in a loving way. This turned him into a pile of mush and he'd say yes. Sticking out my tongue become my way of saying, "I love you Dad" without even saying it.
I still pull that one to this day!

Another great memory I have is that he always made my Halloween costumes. He got so creative and put so much time into them that it amazed me. He knew it was my favorite holiday and wanted to make me unique costumes. This is one of those examples of how something so little can have such a great impact on your relationship with someone. My father was my hero growing up and I'm really grateful for that.

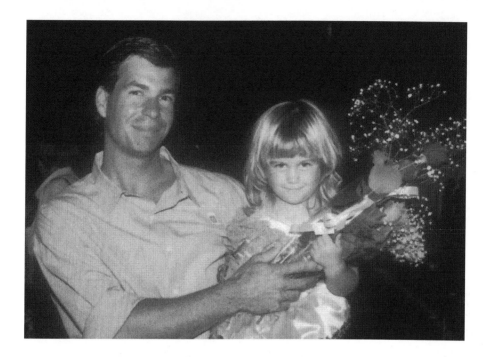

My brother has always been an important part of my life because I knew I was his older sister and he looked up to me. He was without a doubt the cutest little brother I could have ever asked for. I'll never forget when my parents went to find out the gender of the baby at the doctor's office. I was about four years old. I wanted a sister so badly, and was hoping they would say it was a girl. Well, I was truly disappointed when they told me my mom was a having a boy. I'm not sure why I wanted a sister so badly, but I can say I'm glad today that it was a boy!

On the day my brother was born, my father came out of the delivery room to show me my new brother. I wasn't used to what newborns looked like, so I was a little surprised. I even said, "Are you sure that's my brother?" After a few months all of that changed. I fell in love with him and thought he was the cutest baby I had ever seen. His big brown eyes and adorable face was the reason I smothered him with kisses. My parents had to tell me to give him room because I would literally kiss his entire face over and over.

I know there are some people out there who hated having a younger sibling come along and steal their spotlight, but not me. He was my favorite person growing up because he was just so cute and he looked up to me. Sure, there were times when I got annoyed because he followed me everywhere. In retrospect, it was because I was his older sister and he wanted to be with me. Our relationship was very healthy and we got along great. He was and still is my little brother who I want to smother with kisses all the time.

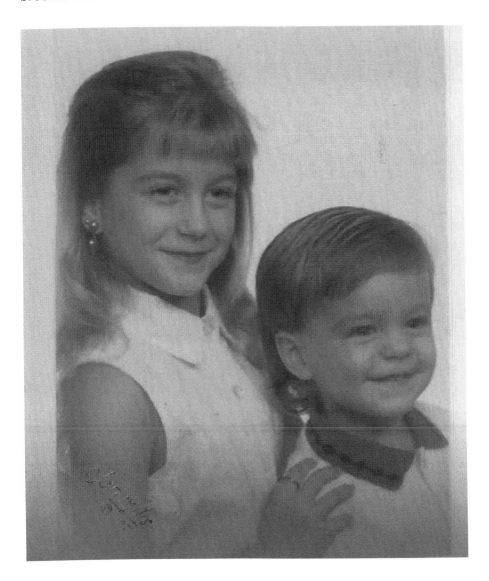

As a child my extended family lived close. I was fortunate enough to have everyone in my family all around me. My father's parents, who I was very close to as a child, lived only fifteen minutes away. My grandparents watched me whenever my parents needed a babysitter. This is very significant because they played an important part in my sobriety.

I loved going to my grandparents' house and getting spoiled. I was the type of kid who would dance around in front of them to get their attention and to show off. I hear many stories from my grandmother about dressing up in her old dresses and pretending to be on stage or in front of a camera. I loved being with them and our relationship quickly grew.

My mom's parents didn't live as close, so I didn't get to see them as often as my other grandparents. When I did see them it was usually on holidays or at my dance recitals. I fondly remember that my grandfather always snuck money to me whenever we were together. As a young kid you don't forget special moments like that. My grandparents never missed any of my dance recitals which meant everything to me. I was very lucky to have them participate in my childhood.

My parents were the type who let me choose what sports I wanted to participate in. They never forced me into anything, but simply asked what my interests were. I told them I wanted to try swimming. They quickly registered me for classes at a local swim school. It didn't take long for me to tell my parents how much I loved swimming. After watching the older kids in the bigger pool, I told my parents I wanted to be on the swim team and they agreed. I joined the team and started competing in local races. I fell in love with competing, at the tender age of five. My first competitive swim victory was in the backstroke. This was my all-time favorite stroke while I was on the team. Ribbons were awarded instead of medals, but getting that blue ribbon was exhilarating and I knew that I wanted more! I started competing in other strokes and closely following every instruction my coach gave me. My collection of ribbons quickly grew and I felt very accomplished.

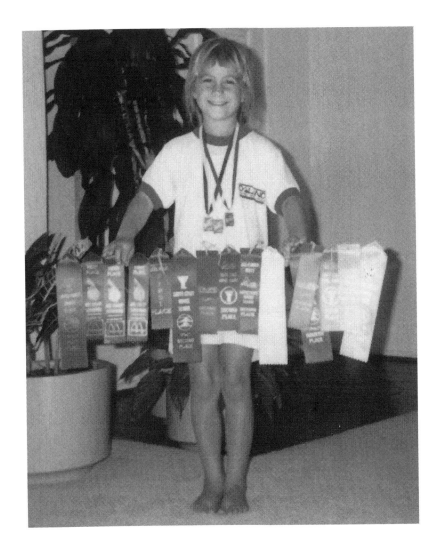

There are many kids out there who could care less about winning at such a young age, but not me. There was something powerful about giving my best shot and getting rewarded for it. Plus, in all honesty, I loved beating other kids. I had my weaknesses in swimming. Both my coach and I knew that freestyle was my weakest stroke. He joked about it because freestyle is usually the easiest stroke for most people. I just shrugged my shoulders, smiled, and told him I just needed to work on it. I always thought positively, even from a young age.

I tried other sports like soccer and I hated it. I tried one game and told my parents that I was never playing again. They told me it wasn't a problem and to try something else. I looked at my mom and said, "I want to be in commercials." At that time my mom had never been involved in the acting industry, so she had to do a lot of research on how to begin.

The first step was getting an agent to represent me. Sounds easy right? It was the complete opposite of easy. We had to send numerous pictures to several agencies in order to get an interview for consideration. Fortunately, I caught the eye of one talent agency in Hollywood who wanted me to audition for representation. She sent the commercial lines to me, so I could practice them beforehand.

As I mentioned before, I wasn't a shy kid, but this was new territory for me. I practiced in front of my parents many times before that audition, to be comfortable with my lines. My mom told me if I messed up the lines to just keep going. I said, "Okay, but I'm not going to mess up. I have the lines memorized." Memorizing the lines wasn't the hard part. Being in front of a stranger and pretending I was in front of a camera was.

Thankfully the agent was very sweet, so I was very comfortable with her. She looked at me and asked me if I was ready. I nodded my head and said, "Yes." I began, got lost in the lines, and forgot my nervousness. I thoroughly enjoyed reciting the lines. When I finished she told me that it was an easy decision for her to represent me. I was ecstatic to hear this!

This opened my eyes to a whole new world. After securing an agent I had to get headshots taken to bring to auditions. My father took me to a professional photographer. I loved getting dressed up and being in front of the camera. Every picture showed how much I enjoyed it.

Once I had my headshots I could start auditioning for jobs. My first audition was for a Rice Krispies commercial. My dad and I drove to

Hollywood. We arrived at the audition; I received my sides, which is another term for lines. I only had one really simple line to memorize, "My cereal goes snap, crackle, pop!" When my name was called I went with two other kids to a room with the casting team and a camera. I spoke my name and then my line. Even though it was only one line I had so much fun doing it. They thanked me and told me that if they wanted a call back they would be contacting me later that day. I never got a call back but knew I still wanted to act. I tried not to get discouraged.

To improve my acting skills, my parents registered me for classes. Every Saturday I went to the Young Actors Space for an hour-long acting class. There were only six students in the class, including one of my dance buddies from Nickelodeon, Amanda Bynes. There was so much talent in that one class and I learned a lot from it.

With the acting classes and numerous hours at auditions, I didn't book many jobs. In the acting industry a lack of job bookings didn't equate to a lack of talent. It usually meant I wasn't quite right for a specific part. My agent told me not to take it personally that I didn't book a job. I had to learn to accept rejection. It's a blunt and harsh industry to be involved with, but at the time I didn't care.

I booked a few jobs here and there but nothing so significant as to keep me out of school and from having a normal childhood. The driving hours, money, and time with dance class became too cumbersome. My parents told me to make a choice between acting and dance. This was a very easy decision for me and I chose dance in a heartbeat. Although, I was disappointed I couldn't maintain both, I understood why and never held it against my parents. I knew how time consuming it was and I was ready to move on with dance and just focus on that.

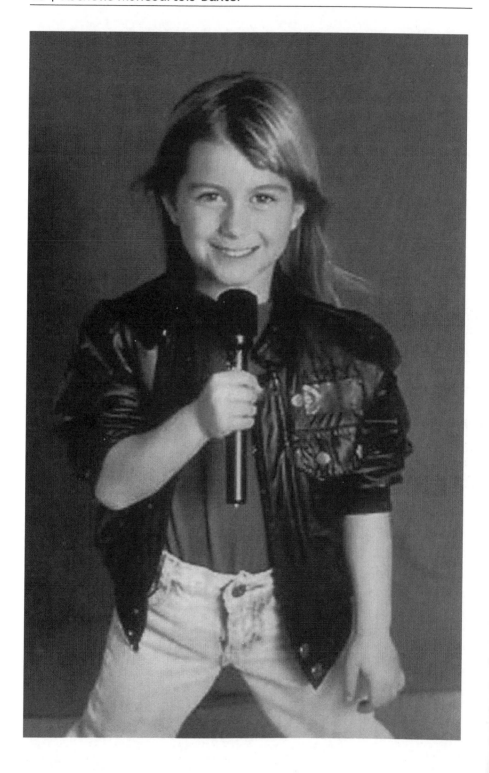

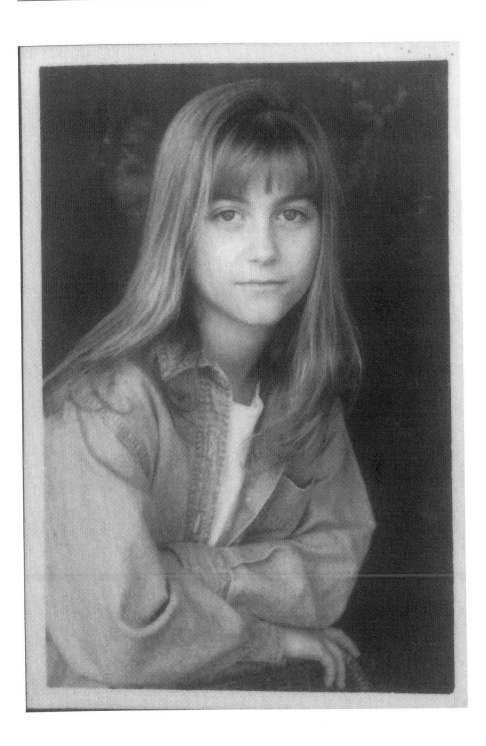

My childhood consisted of being involved in sports, school, family, and spending time with my friends. Nothing in my childhood was out of the ordinary or traumatic. I never had issues with my family, never dealt with death, and was surrounded by great people in general.

As I mentioned before, a lot of people firmly believe that all alcoholics or addicts came from a dysfunctional or unstable household. I am one of the few alcoholics who grew up in a loving, stable, and very healthy environment. People need to understand that alcoholics and addicts come from all different backgrounds and all have different stories leading up to their addiction.

"Growing up Alcoholic," only meant that the disease was hibernating and waiting for the right time to strike. I went through a series of events that led to my alcoholism later in life.

Chapter 2
Dance is my Passion

My favorite memory as a child is the day my parents took me to a doctor because I was slightly pigeon-toed. Little did I know that this doctor appointment would be a life changing experience for me. They took me to the doctor to find out how to correct the problem. The doctor told my parents that the best way to correct my feet would be through ballet which would teach me to turn my toes outward. I wasn't sure if I would like ballet, but said I would try.

My parents immediately signed me up for a trial ballet class and hoped for the best. When I entered that first ballet class, I had no idea that my life would be forever changed. I vividly remember the dance room and the classical music. I thought it was a very cool thing. After that class was over, I had fallen in love with dance.

Since I loved the first class, my parents registered me for weekly ballet and tap dance lessons. Saturdays became my favorite day of the week because I knew I would be going to dance class. I had my first dance recital at three years old and can remember the exhilarating feeling of being on stage in front of a crowd. I loved it! My dancing skills were not yet developed because of my age, but that changed with practice and time. I continued to take ballet and tap classes until I was about seven years old.

During that time, my studio also held dance camps over the summer to keep students involved with dance and the studio. The dance camps were always two weeks long and we put on a performance at the conclusion of the camp. Each camp had a different musical or play. When I was five years old the camp I attended had "The Little Mermaid" theme. The lead role of Ariel had a solo part that I wanted to sing. Since I was so young I was afraid that I would not be considered for the lead role. Because of my past acting experience and my love of being in front of the camera, I had the confidence to go directly to the camp director and ask for an audition. I auditioned and got the part. I was so excited to tell the news to my parents. This clearly illustrated how I was able, at a very young age, to go after something I wanted.

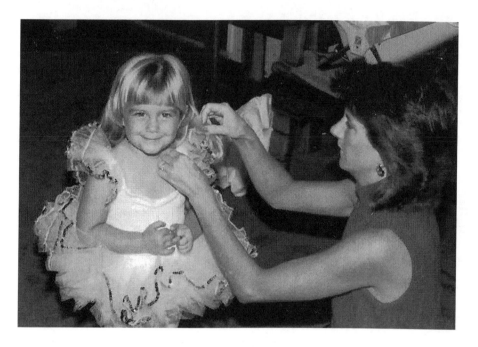

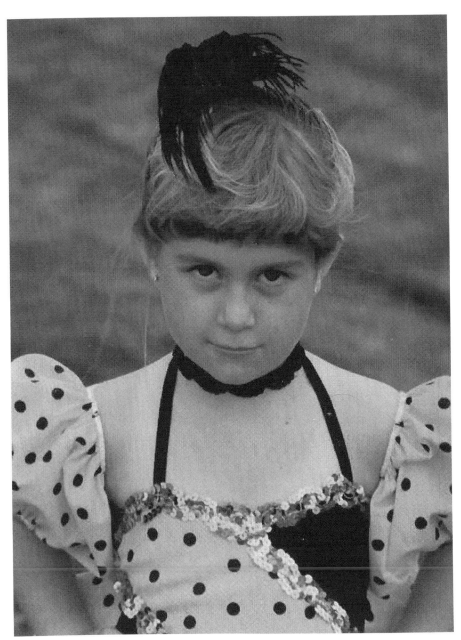

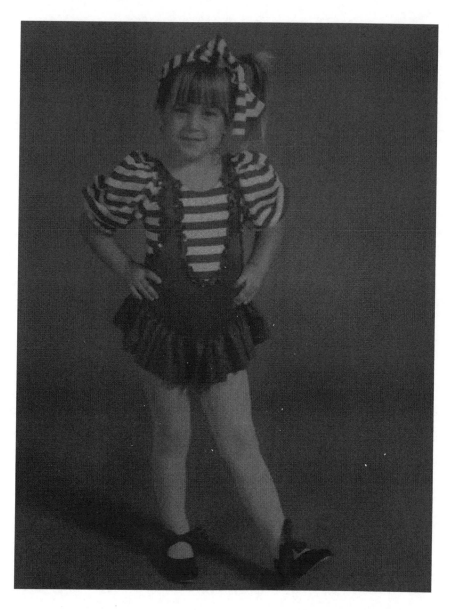

At age seven I noticed that there was another type of dance class called jazz but it was only for students age eight and older. I told my mom that I wanted to try it because it looked like fun and I thought I liked the style better than tap and ballet. My mom told me that if I wanted to take the class I would have to ask the owner myself. I asked and was granted an audition for the jazz dance company. Once again, my previous experience gave me the confidence and courage to do this. I auditioned and was accepted.

This opened a whole new dance world to me and marks a moment when it truly became my passion in life. I began taking hours of required ballet, jazz, lyrical, tap and hip-hop classes.

Jazz and hip-hop quickly became my "thing." When I took jazz or hip-hop classes I gave it one hundred percent and made sure I stood out from the other girls. I really wanted to perform a solo and doing this would greatly increase my chances of achieving this.

The owner did notice me and asked if I was interested in performing in solos. I quickly said I was very interested! She told me that I could do two, including a lyrical and a hip-hop solo. The fact that I was only eight years old made this offer even more amazing. I had to be capable of filling the entire stage with my performance alone. I knew this wouldn't be easy but wanted it badly enough to work hard to accomplish it.

I was given my choice of instructors to choreograph my dance routine; I chose the instructor who stood out for her dancing ability and performance skills. I knew if I wanted to be the best I would have to train with the best, so I walked right up to her and asked her to be my choreographer. She told me that she would love to work with me which was very exciting.

The relationship with my dance instructor was very significant because she was the one who made me the dancer I am today. She taught me to never say, "I can't do that." She told me to trust every dance move she gave me. This set up a lifetime practice of knowing that I could do anything as long as I tried.

My first solo performance was extremely memorable. I took the stage, looked out at the audience and knew that every eye was on me. To an eight year old, this was a very intense feeling accompanied by great pressure. As soon as the music started I forgot about it all and gave them my best performance. I didn't win first place, but I felt like a winner when I finished my performance. That was the moment that I knew I wanted to compete and not just dance for pleasure. My competitive side was beginning to emerge.

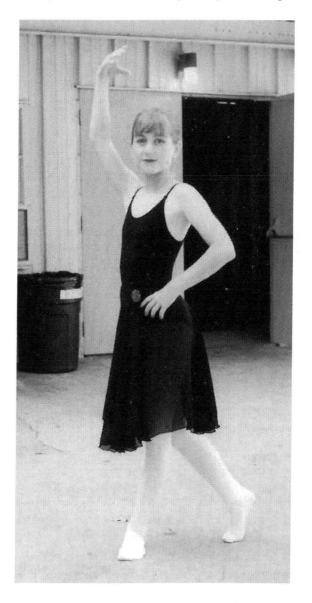

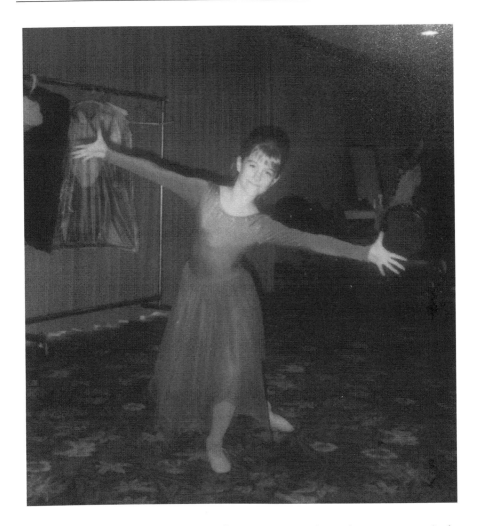

My relationship with my dance instructor continued to grow and she started calling me her little "protégé." We became so close that I asked her to choreograph two other competition solos for me. This is when my performance skills really improved. She taught me how to capture the audience's attention and make myself stand out from other dancers. She taught me how to freestyle and show facial expressions while dancing. She was my dance role model.

The long, hard hours of dance practice continued until I felt as though I didn't have enough energy to make it to class one night. I told my mom how I was feeling. Taking off one class didn't improve how I felt so my mom took me to a doctor to find out why. A simple blood test confirmed that I had the infectious mononucleosis virus. I was only in the third grade and didn't understand the impact it would have on me. I needed to stop dancing for weeks or maybe months in order to properly recover. I cried and worried about missing so much practice time.

After three months my doctor gave me the clearance to return to dance class. I wasn't eager to return because I was concerned about all the time and practice I had missed while home recovering from the virus. When my mom took me to the studio for my first class back, I told her I wanted to quit dance. This shocked her because she knew how passionate I was about dancing. She left me crying in the car and went inside to get the studio owner. I sat in the car and thought about how far behind I would be. I was terrified. The owner came out to the car and told me that I had too much talent to quit. After some thought and trepidation, I made the decision to go back through the studio doors and begin where I had left off. I give total credit to my ever faithful mom and the studio owner for helping me make the right decision that day.

The dance studio started putting me in dances that were meant to be performed in competition. My first group dance was a jazz piece to "One, Singular Sensations," from Chorus Line. My favorite dance instructor was one of two choreographers for the competition dance. My relationship with her grew even stronger during these rehearsals and dance classes. I admired her and wanted to imitate her dance style. I listened to every single correction she gave me because I knew it would make me a better dancer. My hard work paid off because I was placed at the front of this dance piece. Choreographers do this to make the best dancers visible to the audience.

Months passed and we were prepared to compete as a group. This particular dance competition we were going to was one of the best-known in Los Angeles, California. The thought of this didn't make me nervous but rather excited! This dance competition was a com-prehensive convention where I got to take dance classes from various instructors. At the end of the day I prepared to perform.

While I was stretching I noticed that the other group from our studio had some dancers that I didn't recognize. I was introduced to one girl in particular so I watched her performance. Little did I know then that she would become a very good friend and play a significant role in my life. My relationship with her became a huge part of my dance story.

On the last day of the weekend, scholarship auditions were held. These auditions had three levels: beginner, intermediate, and advanced. I was considered a beginner and knew that I would really have to shine to be noticed. My competitive personality compelled me to the front row nearest the instructor. While I practiced the steps I gave one hundred percent and made sure to make eye contact with the judges. I knew that I had gotten their attention but still needed to complete the audition.

When it was time for the audition, I was not placed in the front row. I was afraid that I would not be noticed by the judges so I slowly made my way to the front as the dance progressed. At the end of the dance there was a thirty second period called "freestyle" where I was able to showcase all my best moves. As an added bonus I winked at one of the judges with whom I had eye contact. This small gesture became my trademark for scholarship audition tryouts. None of the other dancers had thought to add this so I knew that it would make me stand out from the others.

At the conclusion of the auditions we were taken into a huge ballroom to announce the winners. I was not nervous at all as I knew that I had performed exceptionally well and was confident that I would win. I did win and it became the first time that I had my name announced publicly. The excitement was overwhelming but I loved it! The feeling of being victorious was something I wanted to repeat.

With a first big dance win under my belt, I wanted to take it to the next level and audition for a dance agent. I had previous experience with an agent for acting so was accustomed to traveling to Hollywood with a few hours' notice to audition to book a job. I loved acting but I loved dance even more and wanted to pursue an agent.

My mom helped me find an open casting call with one of the biggest dance agencies at the time. An open casting call meant anyone could go audition. I told her I wanted to go. I was only ten years old and hadn't done a solo freestyle in front of three judges. I was intimidated but carefully observed the kids who went before me and just told myself to go and have fun with it.

They called my name to step out on the floor to audition. I knew that I needed to do something unique to increase my chance of winning. I put on the flannel shirt that was tied around my waist. Once the music began I busted out a few hip-hop moves, removed the shirt, tossed it to the side and with good eye contact, gave my trademark wink. They told me on the spot that they wanted to represent me. I jumped up and down with excitement. It felt like another "win" and I couldn't get enough of that feeling. I set out to get an agent and I had made it happen.

Now that I had an agent, I had to go get new headshots and start the audition process just like I had done with acting. The only difference was that I had to learn dance routines with a group and then freestyle at the end. This made the auditions last longer and so became more time consuming. I enjoyed dance auditions more than acting because I felt like it came naturally to me. I never really got nervous about dance auditions like I had with acting. I always told myself that if I ever made a mistake I could just freestyle. In acting auditions, a mistaken line was very obvious. I didn't book jobs non-stop, but I did book a few here and there. I never took it personally and just kept moving forward after each audition. Most of my dance instructors had experience with dance agents and told me if I got rejected to just move on. Mentally that sounded easy to do but for a perfectionist, it was difficult.

I didn't know this at the time but being a perfectionist was the beginning of my alcoholism. Perfectionism was a characteristic that started developing and really affected me in a negative way. I wanted to book every audition I attended but that was impossible. When I was younger it was easier to move on after being rejected but later in life that changed.

Perfectionism is something that I had in common with my best friend at the dance studio. We quickly became close and were soon inseparable. Our common perfectionism made us both want to be the best dancer possible and we were willing to work hard to achieve this. We knew that there was a time to be serious and a time to have fun. We tried not to be too hard on ourselves, but the perfectionism made it difficult. I encouraged her to audition for the dance company so we could dance together more. She auditioned, made it and we became joined at the hip.

The name of our dance studio was "Bobbie's School of Performing Arts." We quickly became known as the "Bobbsie Twins." We coordinated our outfits for class and pretended to be sisters. We did everything together except attend the same middle school. We loved being together as much as possible. We were the perfect dance duo. She loved ballet and I loved hip-hop. Her dance technique was very advanced for her age. She excelled in ballet and lyrical, while I excelled in jazz and hip-hop. Our dance styles were a perfect mixture of styles and performance. We decided that we wanted to do a dance duo together.

Choosing an instructor to choreograph our dance was a difficult decision. Over the years we had both gotten close to a few of the instructors at the studio, so had several from whom to choose. We made our choice and began the task of performing a lyrical dance duo together. We both worked extremely hard because we both wanted to win more than anything. Our dedication at such a young age was pretty incredible.

This is when my dedication and commitment trait started to form. Both of these traits are very important to me to this day. Without them we wouldn't have performed as well as we did. While we were getting ready for the competition I saw how nervous my best friend was. I told her we just needed to go out, do our best, and hope it was good enough to win.

Having a perfectionist personality played a big part in my alcoholism. Since my best friend shared that trait, we were constantly trying to perfect every move and every step so that our finished dance was flawless and clean. One technical move, called a "ponche," was the opening move in our dance. We practiced it and nailed it every time. When we performed the dance, I let my nerves get to me and I slightly fell out of the move at the very beginning of the dance. It would be my first taste of defeat and it felt like the worst thing that had ever happened to me. It caused me to be two counts ahead of my partner which spells disaster for a duo performance. Thankfully I regained my composure, continued, and finished strong. After exiting the stage, I apologized to my friend for my mistake. She told me not to worry about it and move on. It was a small statement but had a great impact on me.

That was one of many dances we performed and competed with each other. We continued to take almost every single dance class and competition piece together. Since we were both at the same level dance-wise, we got placed into dances with older girls. This is not the usual policy for our dance studio. The exception was made if a choreographer decided that a younger student had the ability to keep up with the more advanced level of dance moves and performances. This is not something we asked for, but our dedication and hard work was noticed and resulted in many invitations to move up to these higher level dances. We were pretty excited to be asked and always agreed to participate. We had a strong belief in our talent and work ethic and knew we could keep up with the older girls.

Although we were competing at the higher level dance competitions, we were still required to take quite a few hours of classes at our age level. Then at the end of the season in June, there would be dance recitals. It was a favorite time with the dancers because recitals were meant to be fun without the pressure of winning. My family was always there supporting me at every recital. I especially liked the end-of-the-year recitals because I was able to hone my technique and performance skills without the nervousness associated with competition.

During the many hours of dance classes, my relationship with my favorite instructor continued to grow. I took every single class she taught because I wanted to be just like her. When I watched her dance I made sure my moves and facial expressions matched hers. She started taking me to Hollywood to attend some dance classes at a studio called "Edge" which I was familiar with because I had won a scholarship to attend there.

These dance classes were full of very talented dancers and I was one of the youngest students. My teacher told me to stand in the front and center. I was thankful for my lack of shyness because this could have been a very intimidating experience for a ten year old. I had complete trust in my teacher so I followed her instructions implicitly. The instructor for the class noticed me and kept me in front the entire class. I felt very proud to be noticed by someone with such status. After class I went over and thanked her and she told me to always stand in front because I had too much talent to be hidden in the back. I took to heart this very powerful suggestion.

There was one other instructor who really inspired me. He was my first male dance instructor and had great talent. I was about eight years old when I took a hip-hop class he was teaching. His dance moves were amazing and he quickly became a favorite of mine. I always took the front and center position in his classes to be sure that he noticed my talents. I told him that hip-hop was my favorite style of dance and that I looked forward to his classes. His instructions and classes played a large part in my dancing career. I will always remember the time he told me I had something special when I performed. I questioned this and he told me that when I performed my smile and presence were attributes that I should never lose. This made a lasting imprint upon me.

As a young kid my mind was like a sponge and I absorbed every bit of information possible. Whenever a teacher instructed me, critiqued me, or corrected my technique, I listened and learned. I wanted to learn everything I could from people I admired. When my teacher critiqued me, I quietly listened because my goal was to be a great dancer like her. She reminded me that I would never be perfect but to work hard to be the best I could be.

My dance world changed drastically when I was in middle school. The owner of the studio approached my best friend and I with a look on her face that told us it wasn't good news. She told us that she had to let my favorite teacher go. I started crying and couldn't speak. I felt my world come crashing down because I had thought her to be the best teacher at the studio. I knew that my dance world would not be the same without her.

I walked out of the room feeling very angry, sad and practically lost. Every dance routine I knew was from her. Whether it was placing first, winning four dance scholarships, or trying new tricks I thought were impossible, she molded me into her own little protégé and I was extremely grateful for that. I didn't know how the rest of my dancing career would turn out without her, but I knew I had to keep dancing.

I continued with my hard work and endless hours of dance practice without her guidance. Not having her as my instructor was difficult, but thankfully there were other instructors I was fond of and admired. Out of all the things I learned from her, the most important was to be myself, try new things, never say "I can't", and not to strive for perfection.

Chapter 3
High School Years

"You can do anything you put your mind to," is a motto I live by daily. In retrospect, I realize that everything I did was in accordance with this motto. Achieving straight A's and winning first in competitions were goals I desired, went for and achieved. That is how drinking was for me. If I wanted to drink, I did it in spite of the consequences.

Everything started to change for me as a pre-teen adolescent. I started to notice my body changes which were significant for a young girl on the brink of womanhood. I had always been on the smaller size for my height and weight but things started to change for me in the eighth grade. I began comparing myself to my friends who were a size "0" even though I was only a size "1" which seemed so much larger by comparison. I began to develop signs of an eating disorder at this time.

I knew that I wanted to change how I looked so I began to pack smaller lunches and eventually worked up to eating only a protein bar for lunch. This was not the proper nutrition for a growing, active, young woman. I began to count calories and fat grams without any knowledge of what I was doing. I lost weight and some of my friends took notice but didn't say anything about my new eating habits. I was never completely anorexic but it did eventually segue into a full blown eating disorder. Looking back I see that this was part of the addiction that would eventually lead to my alcoholism.

Since I lived in Moorpark, California, I was supposed to go to the local high school but preferred to go to Thousand Oaks High School in Thousand Oaks because all of my studio dance friends attended school there. I knew that it would greatly increase my chance of attending school there if I could make their dance team. I registered for the dance team tryouts and began working on my audition. My past experience with auditions gave me the confidence to simply choose some music and then perform my audition solo piece in freestyle with my trademark wink to leave a lasting impression.

After the auditions I was anxious to find out the results. My best friend and I went a few days later to see if we had made the team and were ecstatic to find out that we had! Being part of a high school dance team was going to be quite different from our experience with the dance studio. We were required to be at the school at 6:30 a.m. Monday through Friday. There were also after school classes and rehearsals most days of the week, dance studio classes and my academic homework to complete. The schedule proved to be too much for me so I had to make the tough decision to quit the dance company and focus on the high school dance team. I would still attend the regular, weekly dance studio classes. This added up to about ten to twelve hours per week. I felt in order to be the best dancer possible I needed these practice hours.

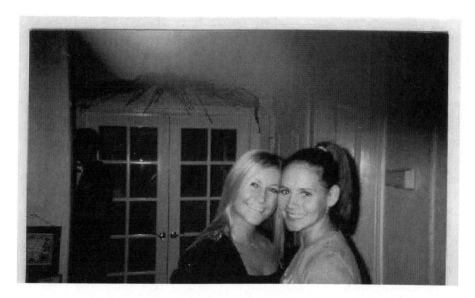

Attending Thousand Oaks High school was not at all like going to a new school where I didn't know many people. I had attended schools in Thousand Oaks, played softball and had friends from my dance studio. I developed a closer friendship with two friends from elementary school and softball. I was happy to be reunited with them and to renew our friendships. They were both smart, pretty all around good kids. They introduced me to their friends from middle school and they soon became my friends. My circle of friends was slowly increasing.

My new friends were an eclectic mix of hard core jocks, cheerleaders, dancers, and athletes from soccer, softball and water polo. We were considered the "popular" kids and none were into drugs or heavy drinking which wasn't a very popular thing to do back then. I knew I had chosen a solid group of teenagers and I liked all of them. Being connected to them truly helped me love my high school experience.

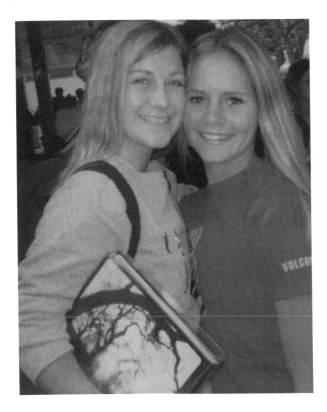

As I continued with the school dance team, my best friend and I were asked to perform solos for an upcoming competition. The head dance coach informed us that this was not the usual policy for freshman students but was confident that we could handle it. We were thrilled! I chose a sexy jazz piece and she went with a lyrical piece because those were our greatest dance strengths and would give us our best performances.

Meanwhile, the atmosphere at the dance studio was changing to the point that I felt invisible during my weekly classes. I felt like I was being ignored by the same teachers who had loved me, encouraged me to stand front and center, and to lead warm ups across the floors. The other students seemed to copy this behavior by being distant and acting as though they were above me. I decided that their behavior change was due to me not being a part of the dance company. I guessed they thought I had become a recreational dancer and wasn't serious any more.

My strong personality wouldn't allow me to be treated this way. I wouldn't let someone walk all over me because of my decision to not participate in the dance company. I told my best friend, who wasn't as bold as me, that I was going to place myself in my former position at the front of the class whether they liked it or not. The look on her face was priceless! I was up front for every warm up, across the floor, and routines we learned during class. I wanted to prove that I was above being ignored and that I wouldn't let it get to me. I wanted to be there to dance and that was the bottom line.

I continued the endless hours of practice with the school dance team. One of my favorite activities was performing for the entire school at rallies where I danced as though I was on stage before millions of people. I was exhilarated when performing this way because I could work on my performance skills and become a better dancer. I was always extremely focused on being noticed whether at a school rally or in dance class for a guest dance instructor. I added special tricks to routines or was first to raise my hand to volunteer to go up front. I knew that I would need to be aggressive in order to be noticed or to book a dance job. Aggressiveness is quite different from arrogance which is something I had to deal with in the dance industry. This can be intimidating to some people but not to me. I just ignored it and danced my heart out every day while enjoying four years of high school.

Even though I had a busy schedule with dance, I still did normal teenage activities such as hanging out at friends' houses, going to the mall and talking on the phone for hours about nothing. I had two very close girlfriends that I spent the most time with; I was the dancer, one played softball, and the other had her own interests. This didn't keep us from spending quality time together and as a whole we got along great and never intentionally hurt each other

My first experience with alcohol was pretty low key. My two friends and I went to a friend's house whose parents were out of town. We all thought it would be funny to drink wine coolers and sit in the hot tub all night. I wasn't a "goody-goody" but didn't want to get into trouble and thought that one wine cooler wouldn't be a big deal. I opened one and took my first sip of alcohol. I finished it and had another. I barely felt the alcohol's effects and didn't quite understand what the fuss was all about. I thought it was kind of boring and never really had intentions of drinking again.

Even though my first experience with alcohol wasn't something very exciting or significant, it was the early beginnings of the slow progression into alcoholism. Many alcoholics tell about the craving feeling they experienced with their first taste of alcohol but I never experienced that. For the remainder of my freshman year I didn't think about or take another drink. I was just focused on dancing and enjoying high school with my friends. Everything was going as planned and my world was drama free, peaceful, fun, and full of activities until one morning at school dance team practice.

I woke up that morning, brushed my teeth, and got ready for school and dance team practice just like any other day. I arrived at class and waited with my best friend for our coach to arrive. Suddenly another dance team member started screaming in my face. It came out of nowhere and I was totally caught off guard since I had known this girl and her sister for many years and considered them both friends. The older sister accused me of elitism because I was always being placed at the front during class and that being "popular" didn't mean anything to her. It was typical high school drama but it was the first time I had felt personally attacked. Her accusations were completely false and I told her so. I walked away toward our dance room with my best friend and began to cry. This was another significant event because I had never cried in front of a friend and she questioned this. I told her I was in shock and had felt attacked. She told me to brush it off, ignore my attacker, and dance my heart out during practice. I was embarrassed at my show of emotions but still wiped my tears, walked into class, and acted like nothing had happened. I wanted to be the stronger person and not show any weakness or retaliate.

This show of emotions was another first for me. It was the first time that I had showed emotion in a situation in which I had no control and then had to appear perfect by acting as if it hadn't bothered me. I didn't mention it to my mother because I didn't want her to get involved and cause it to escalate further but it did in spite of my caution. Another night during rehearsal for a school rally in which we had chosen a male partner, my friends and I started chatting. The same girl that had confronted me was also a leader and she sat us out of the routine for talking. I felt as though we were singled out because many other students had been talking. I made the quick decision to take care of the situation so I asked her if I could talk to her outside. Since she was a senior this was a very bold move for a freshman.

With resentment in my heart and not thinking about what I would say I simply told her that I wasn't going to let her ruin my freshman year by treating my friend and me unfairly and that her comments about my popularity had nothing to do with how I was treated during class. She overreacted to my comments and for the first time in my life I felt like using physical violence against someone. My best friend had been observing the situation and noticed my clenched fist. She quickly came over to me, grabbed my fist, and told me this girl wasn't worth a physical confrontation. I took a deep breath, looked at my antagonist, and walked back into the dance room.

As I walked into the dance room, my heart was rapidly pounding, and the other students sensed that something had happened. I smiled and acted like nothing was amiss but deep down I was angry and hurt. When my mom arrived to pick me up she noticed something was wrong and asked me about it. I began to cry and told her what had happened. She asked me who the girl was so I pointed her out. With a motherly instinct to protect me, she got out of the car, walked up to this girl, and told her that her behavior was unacceptable and to stop treating me unfairly. I'll always be grateful to my mom for backing me up and her adult presence did indeed help the situation.

I looked at my mom, thanked her and knew then that our relationship had deepened because she had defended me in my time of need. I had hoped to forget about the whole situation and move forward but it wasn't to be. The tension in the dance classroom remained for the duration of my freshman year. No more words were exchanged because I didn't want another bad situation to occur. I focused on enjoying the remainder of the school year and danced my heart out in order to become the best dancer possible.

Although I thought I was moving forward I held onto resentment over the situation. I wouldn't realize this until later in life. It lasted throughout my entire dance career and the remainder of my high school experience. Holding onto resentment is like waiting for the other person to drink poison. Obviously this is something that won't happen, so I was the one who actually suffered.

As the school year came to a close I reflected on it and decided that it had been a mostly enjoyable journey. The dance team end-of-the-year banquet quickly approached and I had to make a tough decision about my involvement with the school dance team and the dance studio. The long hours of practice and the tension within the school dance team weighed heavily on me so I made the decision to quit and continue with the dance company at the studio. In my heart I knew that I just wanted to compete in the old dance studio competitions. I said goodbye and looked forward to a new chapter in my life and my sophomore year of high school.

I anticipated my transition from freshman to sophomore and moving up in the ranks at school. Although I was back at the studio as part of the dance company and its competition, I felt compelled to try a different extracurricular activity at school. I decided to try out for the cheerleading squad. I already had friendships with most of the girls on the squad so I wasn't intimidated with the prospect of tryouts. Cheerleading tryouts would be different from dance, but I went out, gave it my best effort and was extremely excited when I made the squad. I loved high school and was happy to have a new activity in which to keep me connected.

My sophomore year arrived and I trained with the cheer squad, danced numerous hours at the studio and maintained good grades. I wasn't any busier than a lot of other students and I always made sure to find time for recreation with my friends. High school and dance studio were two separate worlds and I had a different group of friends for each. My friendships with the cheer squad deepened and I enjoyed the social times I had with them. I was still extremely focused on being the best dancer possible so I requested that I opt out of performing the possibly dangerous stunts and instead simply perform the dance part of the routines at the football games. My request was granted by the coach. I thoroughly enjoyed cheering at school rallies, football games and other sporting events. I became close to one girl in particular. She was funny, outgoing, popular, and always fun to be around. I also maintained my close friendships at the dance studio.

My second drinking experience was with my best friend from freshman year. We heard about a snowboarding trip called "Invasion" and received permission from our parents to attend. The trip was poorly supervised and the party began shortly after the bus left our city. The guys on the bus started drinking right away, but my friend, two other girls and I decided to wait. Smoking pot and vomiting occurred in the back of the bus and we laughed at how ridiculous they looked. Once we arrived at the hotel I was focused on the snowboarding instead of the partying. My friend and I wanted to save the drinking for later that night.

After snowboarding for the day, my friend and I decided it was time to start drinking. Since I had already tried wine coolers I wanted to try drinking shots of whiskey. After the first shot I thought the smell was horrible, the taste disgusting, and remember wanting to throw up. Once the alcohol took effect I felt differently. I thought it was fabulous and thought feeling buzzed made everything more fun. I consumed large amounts of pizza but nothing bad happened to me that night. I never got totally wasted nor did I feel like I couldn't stop drinking when I felt I had had enough. I was not visibly intoxicated to others around me, but just the nice, talkative, outgoing girl I had always been.

I had my first bad experience with alcohol during my sophomore year. My parents were out of town and I invited my twenty-one year old cousin to stay with me to keep me company. I also invited a few close friends to come and have a few drinks. I was introduced to Raspberry Smirnoff vodka and clearly remember taking that first drink and loving every moment of it. As the night wore on I continued drinking and having a good time. Before long I wasn't enjoying myself or feeling well and eventually found myself in the bathroom being sick to my stomach. At one point I was so out of it that I grabbed a curling iron instead of a towel and wiped my mouth with it. Both my cousin and I thought it was pretty funny and joked about it for several years.

After this experience with alcohol, I quit drinking for a while because I didn't want to experience the bad effects from being intoxicated. My next experience with a mind altering substance was with marijuana. Some of my friends had tried it but it wasn't really the popular thing to do at the time. I had heard of it and had been around it so my friend and I decided to try it and see what all the fuss was about. We purchased some, tried it and immediately disliked it. It tasted awful, the smell was even worse, and I didn't feel any immediate effects from it. I wasn't interested in trying it again until some friends told me that it needed to be tried a few more times to feel anything. I tried it once more and later regretted this decision. I took a huge hit from a four-foot bong and immediately hated it the moment that I felt the effects. It was without a doubt the worst feeling I had ever experienced. I felt lost and as though I was in a dream that caused me to feel like crying until it was over. I shared my feelings about smoking pot with my friend and vowed to never touch it again.

The two bad experiences with alcohol and drugs didn't detract from my happiness. My friends would describe me as someone who always smiled despite bad circumstances. I was satisfied with my life and loved high school, long hours at the dance studio practicing and rehearsing, and preparing for competitions.

The studio was preparing for a big competition called the New York Dance Alliance. It would be a new competition for me and I knew that there would be some major scholarship auditions at the conclusion of the competitions. I didn't share with anybody that the real reason I was attending was specifically to win my fourth dance scholarship. I was still required to perform a jazz piece number with the dance team. I had a part where I did a trick jump which I nailed every time we rehearsed the number. When it came time to do my part, I jumped perfectly but landed wrong, rolled my ankle and felt practically unbearable pain. I knew that I had to finish so I pushed through the pain and completed the dance. As I exited the stage I began to cry because I was fairly certain that I had broken my foot or ankle. I still managed to perform the scholarship audition. I put on a fake smile, danced with intense pain and gave my signature wink at the end to impress the judges.

While I waited for the announcement of the winners I felt confident that I had won. When they announced my name I couldn't have been more excited to have won my fourth dance scholarship! Winning this competition meant a trip to New York to perform a solo piece. I had never been to New York and was looking forward to going there. I continued dance practices, ignoring the pain, until I couldn't stand the pain any longer. I went to the doctor but had waited too long so my foot couldn't be casted which meant six to eight weeks in a boot. My dream of competing in New York had come to an end and I was devastated. This situation taught me that I had to take responsibility for my actions and not neglect my well-being or there would be consequences.

I had learned from my experience with mono that staying away from the studio during a long rehab would distance me and cause me anxiety upon my return. This time I sat in on every single dance class that I would have participated in if I had not been injured. Although it was hard to watch my peers continue with their classes,

I knew that being there was important to my psyche. After about eight weeks my doctor released me to resume dance classes and didn't experience the anxious return from several years ago.

I didn't let this temporary setback affect my enjoyment in other activities. I wanted to take in every moment of high school and enjoy it all. I didn't want a boyfriend, avoided unnecessary drama as much as possible, and hung out with friends. I was a very happy, friendly and caring teenager. The remainder of the year was filled with academics and good grades, many hours of dance practice, and maintaining healthy relationships with family and friends.

Sophomore year ended, summer quickly flew by, and I began my junior year of high school with some new goals in mind. As a junior I was now eligible to try out for the "song" part of the cheerleading squad. Song leaders were cheerleaders who didn't perform stunts during rallies and football games but performed dances on their own. It was a goal that I was very passionate about because I would be able to perform as much as possible. The tryouts were well within my comfort zone so I was confident that I would make it. I was ecstatic to learn that not only had I made it but three other friends had as well. We were now on the varsity squad and would perform with the senior girls. I was totally serious about my cheer performances, using them to further perfect my dance performance skills. I wanted to be the best and perfect, which as a future alcoholic, was going to present itself as trouble in later years.

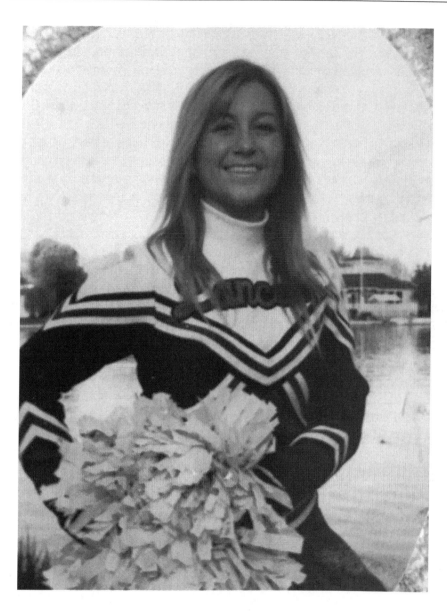

A huge contributing factor to this problem was my admiration of Britney Spears. In her early years I had thought her to be a mediocre performer at best until I saw her "Stronger" video on television. I watched her dance moves, thought her to be amazing and beautiful, and she became my new role model. I watched her videos and memorized the entire dance. I choreographed a dance routine for cheer based on one of her songs and performed it at a rally. When performing I mimicked her moves and was complimented that I danced just like her. Over time I started to incorporate her dance style into more of my routines. I gradually began to take notice of how physically fit she was.

I became more aware of my body image at this time and although I was never overweight, I compared myself to the stick thin images of celebrities and dancers on television and magazine covers. I wanted to have smoking hot abs like them but didn't have a good understanding on how to accomplish this. At 5'2" and 115 pounds I should have been content with my body but the constant comparison to others who were thinner or taller nagged at me. I hid this from everybody including my closest friends. I didn't consider myself fat but rather not perfect looking enough. I began the slow progression toward a major eating disorder and the early beginning of my alcoholism. My perfectionism and over-achievement personality were really starting to emerge.

My junior year continued with endless hours at the dance studio and cheerleading practices, school dances and a few instances of drinking alcohol. I don't remember exactly how many times I drank, but it wasn't a lot. I drank when I attended parties but never got out of control. I drank just like any other "normal" teenager even though, unbeknownst to me, my alcoholism was still progressing.

Another situation at the dance studio occurred and caused great resentment within me. My friend and I had felt like the atmosphere at the studio had improved and we were being treated fairly again until the studio owner approached us just before a dance competition. She quietly told us that she needed to speak to us outside. The presence of another instructor and their tense mood made it obvious that this wasn't going to be a good conversation. The owner told us that she felt as though we were prima donnas because we were always at the front of practices and performances and had won numerous competitions. We were both confused and stunned at this announcement because we felt that they were mistaking our confidence for arrogance.

My friend began to cry so I spoke up and told them that they were incorrect in their assessment, citing the fact that we had been asked and placed in the front by instructors and had earned our places through hard work and dedication. I said that if other students wanted to be like us then they needed to work harder and go into each practice wanting to be the best dancer possible, as I had done. My boldness was a surprise to the owner and instructor. They hadn't expected such a young girl to stand up for herself. My feelings toward the instructor were forever changed after that because I had felt ambushed. My previous admiration of her was greatly diminished and I wondered how this problem would turn out.

After they left us, I looked at my friend and saw how distressed she was. I told her that we needed to go back inside and give the best performance possible despite our wounded feelings. It was at this moment that I realized I was a fighter and didn't want anybody walking all over me and taking away something that I had earned. I worked hard for all of my accolades in dancing and put my heart and soul into every practice and performance. I finished the year at the studio with my head held high. Deep down inside I was still bothered so I talked to my mom about the situation. I decided that I wanted to take my talent and hard work to someone who believed in me and my goals for my dancing. After fifteen years it was time for me to move on, let this door close and look for another one to open.

I was scheduled for oral surgery the summer prior to my senior year of high school. After the surgery I was instructed to only eat liquids or soft foods for several days which caused me to lose about five pounds. I didn't really notice the weight loss until my peers made comments about how great I looked. Instead of feeling grateful for the compliments I wondered what was wrong with me before the weight loss. Had I been overweight? I continued to receive compliments and encouragement to "keep it up." I felt more womanly with my leaner figure and closer to my idea of "perfect."

With my new, lighter figure and increased confidence in my looks, I knew my senior year was going to be fantastic. Unfortunately that wasn't to be. A new coach was hired for our cheerleading squad and was not well liked. She took all the fun out of it and everybody dreaded going to practice. When the usual time arrived to split the squad into cheerleaders and song leaders, our coach surprised us by eliminating the song leaders. I was disappointed to hear this because I had always enjoyed the dance performance part of the song leading squad. Every song leader dropped out and fought to have it returned to the way it was. We lost our battle and my senior cheerleading friends quit leaving only underclass girls on the varsity squad that year. As a teenage girl it felt like the end of the world but I knew I had to move on.

The combined resentment from the dance studio and cheerleading incidents began to fester inside of me. I was never an outwardly emotional female and was used to hiding my emotions until something significant enough occurred to make me speak my mind. I disliked confrontation because I hated drama so it was easier to avoid it altogether. I considered this a strength rather than a weakness.

The two major incidents were traumatic for me but I didn't turn to alcohol because of them. I just stuffed the resentments deep inside of me and tried to move forward to the best of my ability. It was not a healthy thing for me to do but it was the only way I knew to cope with the simmering feelings of resentment. I put on my brave face and signature smile and went on with my senior year.

Since this would be my last year at Thousand Oaks High School I knew I wanted to make the most of it. I decided that I wanted to run for Homecoming Queen since I had never been nominated for Homecoming Princess. I was thrilled when my name was announced as a nominee along with two of my best friends. I had always wanted to be well-liked and I cared about my reputation. I wanted to be a good role model for younger girls. I was so content with just being nominated that I simply enjoyed the process that led up to the elections.

The big announcement was to be made at the Homecoming Football Game and I arrived at the game in a limousine during halftime. As I exited the limousine my name was announced and I waved to the crowd. I was thrilled to be in front of so many people. I loved and lived to perform and at that moment I knew that this was what I wanted to do for the rest of my life but on a larger scale. I wanted to be famous like Britney Spears, hear my name being announced and hear the roar of the crowd as they watched me. I didn't win that night but had an inner victory and a sense that I was destined for a life of performance and fame. I never told anyone about my dream because I thought they would think me crazy. It was a lofty goal and my motto became, "Dream big or go home."

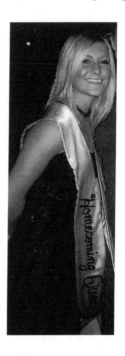

Now that I had a big dream in mind I knew that I needed to get involved in a dance studio to further improve upon my dancing performance skills. I didn't want to go back to my former studio so I set out to find another one. During my search I discovered that my former favorite instructor was teaching close to where I lived. I registered for her dance classes and showed up for my first class. It had been several years since I last saw her but when she saw me in her class she was so excited and introduced me to her class as her little protégé. She requested that I take my former front and center position. We warmed up and began practice. I immediately felt right at home and realized how much I had missed her style, music and our special bond.

Senior year was all that I had hoped it would be. I had great friends, I was back dancing for my original role model, and I was having fun. I never doubted myself and always held the right amount of confidence without being cocky. My dance instructor told me to be a diva on stage but when off stage be just like any other eighteen year old high school girl. It was important to me to be humble. When I performed I wanted to be the best dancer and stand out from the others.

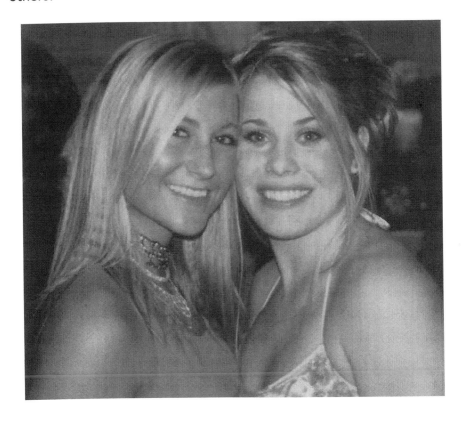

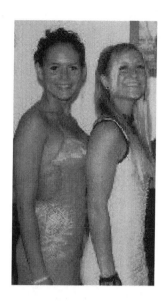 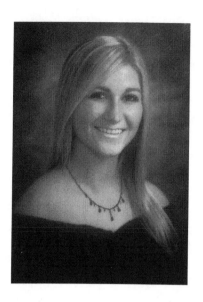

My next experience with vodka was before the Homecoming Dance. I met with my friends before the dance to get ready. My best friend and I thought that it would be fun to drink a little before the dance. We found someone of legal age to purchase the vodka for us and we took a few shots. I didn't want to repeat my previous experience with vodka so I didn't overdrink. I had enough alcohol to get slightly buzzed and had a blast. We danced and enjoyed the evening and when the dance was over I knew I would probably try drinking again but didn't have any overwhelming urge to do so. Those opportunities did arise but I was never the drunk girl at the party. I drank a few shots and then carried on with the fun. Even though my drinking was under control and similar to that of my friends, my alcoholism was slowly progressing.

My senior year was moving along nicely until I awakened one morning not wanting to get out of bed. I didn't feel sick but didn't want to talk to anyone or go to school. This was very atypical of me as I was usually a social butterfly and always wanted to be active and around people. I tried to brush it off but the same thing happened the next morning. I didn't know it at the time but it was the beginning of my depression.

Everything changed for me then. I became very unsocial, didn't want to leave the house or talk to anyone, and my eating habits changed. The depression made me feel like I was mentally out of control so I decided to take control of my eating. I thought that maybe I'd be happier if I were thinner and therefore help fulfill my dream of becoming a famous performer. I obsessed about this until I decided to take action that would lead me down a very dangerous life pathway.

I researched eating disorders and how to hide them from family and friends. I began to eat less and less until I realized that I couldn't function with less calories. I had headaches and felt faint at times so I decided to try a different tactic. I sat down, ate a healthy dinner and then went into the bathroom and forced myself to vomit my dinner. The disgusting part about all this was that I felt good afterwards. I thought that this would help shut out those awful feelings I'd been having. The brief moment of vomiting my dinner did shut off those feelings and I felt like a million bucks. I was relieved and was sure that I had found the cure I was looking for.

I began to vomit after almost every meal and all but eliminated any between meal snacks. The weight came off quickly and people began to notice. It didn't matter if I heard positive or negative comments - I was getting attention because of it. I enjoyed the positive comments on my new thinness and how great I looked. I guarded my secret well and hoped nobody was aware of my eating disorder. Some people may have suspected but kept it to themselves.

My eating disorder was just one symptom of my slowly progressing alcoholism. Depression was the other one that continued to get worse until daily life began to get harder for me to handle. The control I had over my eating was the only thing that made it diminish. As a strong person I didn't see this as a weakness but rather a way to get ahead and ultimately achieve my life goals. All forms of media convinced me that thinner was better and would be my ticket to being that "perfect" female everybody wanted to be. If I had to vomit my way to it then that's what I would do.

I was able to keep my drinking under control throughout my senior year. When graduation arrived there were no parties to attend because my high school had an event called Grad Night and most students opted for this. Grad Night was a trip to Disneyland right after our graduation ceremony and I stayed up all night. I noticed people sneaking alcohol into bras, water bottles and purses. My best friend and I were too afraid to try that so we decided to take some Percocet instead. We had a great time that night and nobody was the wiser about our condition. I didn't like the feeling it gave me and thought it would have been better to drink instead.

In retrospect, my senior year was significant because everything started to change for me. All my peers were talking about college choices and what majors they were considering. I had no intention of attending college because it didn't appeal to me. I still wanted to pursue my dream of becoming a famous performer. At times I felt left out because of my life goal but at the same time I felt my choice was the right one for me. I wanted a different kind of success that others didn't understand. I kept all these thoughts and feelings deep inside of me along with my eating disorder and depression.

Now that my senior year had concluded I spent my summer with my usual group of friends. A friend from dance team and song leading started to hang out almost every single day after we graduated. We wanted this summer to be the best and wanted to go all out. This choice would change my life forever and my drinking would take a turn for the worse.

Chapter 4
Battling My Inner Demons

After high school graduation many of my friends were excited about their journey into adulthood and going away to college to truly find themselves and a future career. I had chosen the life of performance and had dreams of being on the big stage. Just the thought of leaving my parents' home to attend an out-of-town college frightened me. I knew that I wasn't ready to make a move like that. I was content to stay at home, work on my dancing, and begin auditions in order to open doors to bigger things. Little did I know that this would be the beginning of battling my inner-most demons.

My first real big audition after graduation was something I had dreamed about for years. I secured a Laker Girls audition. Laker Girls are dancers that perform at Los Angeles Lakers basketball games. A former dance instructor had been a Laker Girl so I contacted her to help me perfect my technique and be well-prepared for the upcoming audition. During our practices she constantly praised me about my dancing improvement and skills and told me that I wouldn't have any problems making the team. It gave me the confidence I needed to go to the audition and give it everything I had.

My mom went with me to the audition for moral support. When I entered the audition room and saw hundreds of blonde girls waiting, I knew the competition would be tough but I was still confident that I was properly prepared to make the team. The first cut was a basic across the floor combination that I knew I was capable of nailing. I was extremely good at leaps, kicks, and second jumps so knew this would be an easy beginning to the audition. We were split into smaller groups and I made sure I was up front in order to be more noticeable to the judges. I nailed every trick and was confident that I had made it to the next cut so I wasn't nervous in the least bit. I waited for the director to come by me and say "stay" which meant making it to the next step, but instead she said "thank you."

I was stunned and felt like a complete failure. This was by far the biggest rejection I had ever experienced and came as a big blow to my confidence. My dreams of making it as a big star were smashed and I began some pretty serious negative self-talk. Maybe I wasn't skinny enough, or was too short, or hadn't worn enough makeup. I was faced with a situation that was out of my control and I didn't know how to handle it. It felt like my world had stopped. The worst part would be telling everybody back home that I had failed. They all knew how badly I wanted to make it so it wouldn't be an easy thing to do. My mom encouraged me to hold my head high and look to next year's auditions.

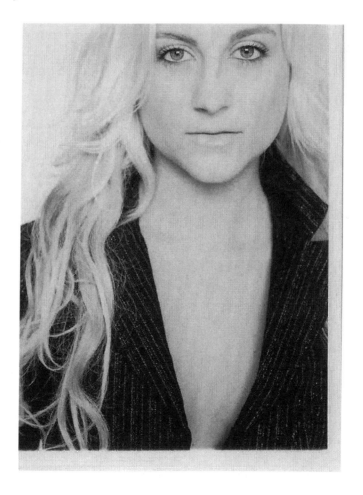

I returned home and focused on the summer fun that my friends and I had planned. We wanted to celebrate the four, wonderful years we had together and I was looking forward to relaxing, hanging out with friends, and attending parties. I didn't want to miss a single party and as the list grew so did my drinking. I attended a party and was introduced to tequila shots. I didn't use a shot glass but grabbed the bottle and took a big swig. The bottle touched my lips, the alcohol hit my throat and stomach, and I felt the instantaneous warming of my body. I felt powerful and alive and nothing was going to stop me from drinking so I could feel this way again.

I continued to chug straight from the bottle, hearing encouragement from my peers to keep going. My brain was loudly telling me that I needed to consume more alcohol. I was having the time of my life and everything was so much more fun, but most importantly, my depressed feelings disappeared. This was the feeling I had been searching for. The alcohol had worked a miracle and all my past bad situations and resentments were gone. As the alcohol flowed throughout my body I felt like my old happy-go-lucky self once more. I continued drinking and experienced my first blackout. I woke up next to my friend and asked her how we had gotten home. I learned later that someone had driven us home without incident and the only souvenir from the party was a terrible hangover. I felt light-headed, dehydrated and nauseous but managed to keep from getting sick to my stomach.

Unfortunately the horrible hangover wasn't enough to deter me from doing the same thing the next night. I chugged tequila straight from the bottle but this time I didn't blackout. I could remember bits and pieces from the evening which didn't include any bad situations. I continued in this manner the rest of the summer. I still enjoyed the euphoric and non-depressed feelings from the effects of the alcohol in spite of the morning-after hangovers. My alcoholism was gradually taking over as I kept equating drinking with the good feelings I experienced under its effects.

My friend and I planned a party at my house when my parents went away for the weekend. We made our guest list and procured alcohol.

Sometime during the party my friend and I discovered a bottle of my dog's medication and thought it would be fun to try some. If I hadn't already been intoxicated my common sense would have told me that it wasn't a good idea. My friend and I each took one shot and felt no immediate effect. When everyone left we went to bed and looked forward to the next day.

I was in and out of a very heavy sleep that night until I was awakened by the ringing of my phone. As I answered it I discovered that it was 5:00 P.M! I had slept an entire day without realizing it. The apparent side effect of the dog's medication had been prolonged sleep. It was the weirdest and scariest feeling I had ever felt and I didn't like it one bit. I told my friend that I was never doing that again. I realized at that moment that I didn't want to try any drug again. The remorse I felt over taking medication didn't keep me from wanting to drink again though.

My parents were still out of town so we wanted to extend our party time one more night. I invited my cousin and a small group of friends for a small get-together. After a few drinks my cousin asked me how I had lost so much weight. My intoxication loosened my tongue and I blurted out that I sometimes vomited after eating. Thankfully she too was intoxicated and didn't take me seriously. We both laughed and returned to the party. I had dodged a bullet for now. I wanted to keep it a secret because I didn't want anybody to know I had insecurities and imperfections.

The rest of the evening continued in the same manner: drinking, talking and just hanging out. After everybody left my friend, who was spending the night, thought we should try the dog's medication again. I wasn't keen on the idea, but she persisted and my alcoholic brain thought another try couldn't hurt anything. The same thing happened as the night before. We took a pill, went to bed and slept until 5:00 P.M. the next day. When I was fully awake and thinking about what I had done I wondered to myself why I had done it. It was part of the insanity behind the alcoholism and its addictive behavior. It caused me to try something once and expect different results the second time.

Once again I was overcome with remorse over taking the dog's medication. I never thought that drinking was wrong because I thought that most teenagers and young adults partied and drank. My remorse turned to guilt when my parents returned home and questioned me about the missing dog medication. I lied and said I didn't know anything about it. This was the first time I had lied to my parents. I was never able to lie because not telling the truth made me laugh and I would be found out. After lying to my parents my guilt increased. As a blossoming alcoholic this would be the beginning of many lies and manipulation. Because I loved my parents I felt awful about lying to them. I vowed to myself to never do that again, a promise I wouldn't be able to keep.

The summer continued in the same pattern of nightly parties and drinking. I was having the time of my life with no cares in the world. I was completely blinded to what was happening to me. The demons from within were slowly rising to the surface. My alcoholism was growing with each sip of alcohol. When the alcohol left my body I returned to a depressed state that disappeared once alcohol flowed through my veins. The cycle would repeat itself on a daily basis.

My cousin continued spending time with me and our relationship grew. One night we threw a party and the only alcohol available was wine. I didn't even like the taste but drank quite a bit of it until I was very drunk. I ran around the kitchen, slipped, went headfirst into the corner of the kitchen cabinet and split open my chin. I didn't really feel any pain but blood was everywhere. My cousin thought I needed stitches but I knew I couldn't go to the hospital with alcohol in my blood. I cleaned myself up and carried on as if nothing happened. This would be the beginning of many bad experiences involving drinking.

I was known as the happy-go-lucky, confident, outgoing girl. The daily smile on my face was a mask that covered up the true feelings inside of me. Deep down inside I wasn't truly happy. The alcohol was only a temporary solution to my depression problem which was getting worse and almost unbearable to handle. The nightly parties gave me a little respite but when the night of drinking was over I was back to feeling depressed again. I even entertained thoughts of suicide which caused me great angst. I couldn't understand why I felt this way. Nothing was really wrong with my life. I had a great family, friends, had just graduated from high school, and had great dance talent. As quickly as it came, I pushed the suicide thought out of my mind and continued to throw back the bottle as much as I could.

One particular night my addictions came to a head after a night of drinking. My friend was passed out on the couch and I was hungry so I found some waffles and ate them. I immediately felt an overwhelming guilt about eating something I wouldn't ordinarily consume, so I ran to the bathroom to throw up. I was unable to make myself vomit and freaked out. In my frenzied thinking I decided to fake a suicide attempt. It was a desperate call for attention. I grabbed the closest knife, made a few small cuts on my wrist, woke up my friend, and she immediately called my parents.

My parents quickly came, picked me up and took me home. Thankfully I wasn't drunk and was completely coherent. I knew what I had done and why I had done it. I cried as my dad carried me into the house because I felt as though I had disappointed my parents and was embarrassed about the whole situation. Regret set in and I realized that it was the desperate feeling of the depression crying out for attention. I thought it was my only option to be able to get out of the deep, dark hole I felt I was in.

When I awakened the next morning I was concerned that people were going to think I was really serious about killing myself and that I had issues. I didn't want people to see me in any way but perfect. My main concern was that my parents were confused and worried sick. My mom asked me about what was happening but I just brushed it off and said that I really didn't want to die and was just depressed for some unknown reason.

This conversation became an open door for a talk with my mom. She told me that she completely understood my feelings because she had gone through depression herself. She told me that there were many options for getting help for how I was feeling. I didn't really want to get help but rather thought it was something that would pass and eventually disappear with time. I managed to convince my mom that I was really okay and didn't need immediate intervention. Alcoholics are master manipulators and I was doing just that without realizing it.

Evading the issue with my mom felt like I had dodged a bullet and gotten away with it. I called my friend and thanked her for her help and went right back to partying and drinking so I could move forward and forget the awful incident. Unfortunately the depression was like a roller coaster where I would feel happy and normal and then had days when I didn't want to get out of bed even though I wasn't hungover. I felt immobile and my brain hurt from thinking. Then there were other times when I burst out crying for no apparent reason. Nothing bad was happening in my life so I was very confused about these over-emotional feelings coming to the surface. I had always been able to keep my feelings and emotions to myself and now they seemed out of control. I wanted to continue with the façade of being the girl who always had a smile on my face when in reality I was hurting on the inside.

Every day became a battle in my mind about why I felt the way I did when there were no apparent external reasons to cause the depression. I had so much going for me and this should have been the happiest season of my life. Instead of getting the help I desperately needed I just tried to brush it off, ignore the nagging blue feelings, and continue with my life as if all was well and normal with me.

Since so many of my friends were going to college, I decided to take a few classes at the local community college in my hometown of Moorpark, California. I registered for ballet, psychology, interior design and speech. I had always enjoyed helping my mom decorate the house so thought that interior design might be an alternative pathway if dancing didn't pan out. With "Plan B" in place I wanted to get back to partying until the summer ended and school began.

As my alcoholism progressed so did my manipulation and lying. My parents were going out of town for a wakeboarding trip and for the first time I told them I didn't want to go. They didn't question this unusual behavior and I found myself home alone and thinking about more nights of drinking. The lie came easier than the ones before which was another sign that I was changing for the worse. I wasn't proud but at the same time didn't really care. All I wanted to do was party and drink. My best friend came over, we called in sick, and began planning our fun week ahead.

The first night's party began with swigging vodka out of a bottle. When the alcohol hit my stomach I immediately felt warmed all over and numb from the emotional pain I had been feeling. I felt beautiful and confident but most importantly I was having a great time. I observed my best friend falling down the stairs, and along with everybody else, thought it was hilarious. As I laughed I told myself that that wouldn't ever happen to me. Then there was a pivotal moment when I realized that I had gone from simply being buzzed to completely drunk with no in between state. This shocked me so I asked everybody to leave so I could go pass out in my bed. I remember thinking I might lean over and vomit all over my sleeping friend. I felt so disgusted by this that I promised myself that I would never drink that much again. This would be a promise easily made and more easily broken over and over.

I woke with the early morning sun and felt absolutely awful. I leaned over to check on my friend and she was completely passed out. I knew I should get up and shower but felt an overwhelming depression and my entire body hurt. I forced myself out of bed, showered and thought about the previous night. I asked myself why I had drunk so much and why I was feeling so miserable the morning after. I decided not to dwell on it, put on my fake smile, and go awaken my friend. I called her name and shook her but she was unconscious. I made sure she was breathing and let her continue to sleep. I didn't know at the time that I would become that "morning after" girl in a few short months.

When my friend finally awakened and became coherent, we discussed what had happened. We both missed the seriousness of the situation and laughed it off as a hilarious experience. I shared with her that I had almost blacked out from the excessive alcohol consumption and again laughed it off. We didn't think that our behavior was any different from any other eighteen year old and that it was just harmless fun. What I couldn't see was that I was slowly becoming "that drunk girl" I never wanted to be.

The memory of the night before and morning after quickly faded and we made plans for another party that night. I invited the same people from the night before and some of my closest high school girlfriends. I wanted to spend as much time with them as possible before they left for college and it had been awhile since we drank together. Our source bought us our alcohol which included beer this time. I started off with a few beers, loosened up, and began reminiscing about our high school days. We discussed one girl in particular that my friend and I weren't fond of because I found out that she was telling others that I was bulimic. I distanced myself from her but held onto resentment over the situation. The alcohol brought up all the intense feelings of betrayal and I knew I had to do something about it.

I suggested that we drive over to her house and confront her in person. A friend who hadn't started drinking was the designated driver and we headed over to her house. We laughed all the way there. When we arrived I called her on the phone and asked for a face-to-face conversation which she refused. This angered me and I began saying things to her that I wouldn't normally say. The conversation got so heated that my friends made the decision to leave to prevent me from getting out of the car and doing physical harm. I felt so angry that the situation wasn't resolved that I grabbed the vodka bottle and started chugging right there in the car. The alcohol immediately worked by numbing these strong, angry emotions, and I returned to the party determined to have a good time.

When we returned to the party, the beer gunning resumed until I reached a full drunken state. The party was winding down and someone who had had too much to drink felt good enough to drive home. I felt otherwise so I suggested that she spend the night and drive home in the morning. She refused my invitation and that set me off. The combined effect of the turbulent evening and excessive alcohol consumption set me off and I began yelling hurtful, angry, out-of-control words. I got so angry that I made a fist and punched a wall. My friends who had not seen this type of behavior from me were shocked but chalked it up to the drinking.

One friend in particular pulled me aside as she was leaving and told me that she missed the girl I used to be. I was too drunk to even take this to heart. This would be my first "Dr. Jekyll, Mr. Hyde" episode. This meant that I drank so much that my personality completely changed and I exhibited behavior that was angry, insulting, and aggressive. I couldn't imagine what my friends thought that night. The alcoholism was slowly making changes within me even when I wasn't drinking. There were changes to me emotionally, physically, and mentally. Unfortunately I was so blinded by the alcohol that I couldn't see it at the time.

The following morning I knew I had to make an apology to my friend for my insanely unfriendly behavior. Without thinking I picked up my cell phone, called her and apologized profusely for my outrageous behavior the previous night. To my surprise she accepted my apology at face value and at that moment I knew that I had a true friend who really cared about me. With emotions overflowing I began sobbing so hard that I could hardly get any words out. The words stumbled from my lips about my deep depression, struggling to get out of bed in the morning, and how drinking made it all go away. She was shocked at my display of emotions because this was the first time she had heard me cry in the four years she had known me. She knew then that there was something seriously wrong with me and she quickly offered to be there for me.

This was the first time that I had ever opened up to someone about how badly I had been feeling. I was finally baring my soul and found that instead of rejection I found acceptance and true friendship. It felt as though a huge weight had been lifted off my shoulders because now it wasn't only my secret but something shared with a friend. I'm forever grateful for that candid moment and the acceptance that I felt. I was able to get up off the floor, wipe away my tears, and thank my friend for caring.

As the summer progressed, so did my drinking. It was a vicious cycle of waking, going to work, and then partying and drinking at night. I was also still battling with my struggle with bulimia. If I had a chance to vomit my food, I did. It wasn't a daily occurrence but progressing nonetheless. It began with once a week to a few times a week. I covered up the sound of me throwing up by pretending to take a shower. The secrecy around this was a different kind of high for me. College classes were quickly approaching and I wanted to look my best on campus. I told myself that the start of classes would be the end of partying and the beginning of getting serious about my future. My first class was interior design which I thought would be something that interested me. After the first class I knew that I already hated college, wasn't the least bit interested in interior design as an alternate career to dance performance, and was looking forward to my afternoon ballet class and attending a drinking party.

I left campus and hurried to my ballet class. My best friend was taking the same class. As we changed into our ballet outfits my friend began staring at me. I questioned this and she told me that I looked really skinny. I took this as a compliment because skinny meant beautiful and perfect to me. I shrugged it off, not wanting to tell her the real reason behind my weight loss. As class began I noticed that I was very low in energy. I had only eaten grapes that day to cut down on calories. The alcoholism and bulimia were both progressing. It became a double whammy for me because I was still battling the bouts of severe depression. It was hard to imagine going through the rest of my life this way.

I told myself that if I wasn't skinny, I couldn't be happy. I was in full pursuit of that "perfect" image and body. I compared myself to the celebrity magazine covers and wanted to look like that. I was prepared to do whatever it took to achieve it and thus attain true happiness. College continued and my drinking became worse. I began going to classes hungover and low in energy from my eating disorder. I didn't like any of the classes I was taking so didn't care about coming to class with a clear mind. Focusing sober was difficult so I wasn't concerned about focusing with a hangover. The demons of addiction were slowly creeping up on me waiting to destroy my life at any moment.

My weight loss became a mind game for me. I looked in the mirror and still saw an imperfect body image that was still in need of more weight loss. To those around me I looked alright on the outside but my insides were suffering. People were noticing my thinness so I thought that more weight loss would make me look even better. I began to vomit more frequently and intensely. I was eventually able to vomit without sticking my finger down my throat. I could just make it come up on its own. My esophagus, teeth, and stomach lining were all beginning to suffer. My electrolyte balance was also suffering and caused irregular heart rhythms. The drinking added to this problem and I was at an even greater risk for a heart attack. I was totally oblivious to this at the time.

Another problem I had was waking up in the morning so dehydrated that I could barely get out of bed to get the water I needed. My muscles ached from lack of proper nutrition and hydration. I attributed this to being hungover instead of the bulimia. I needed to look perfect and that was all I could think about. I looked to ways to lose even more weight and turned to laxatives. I took a pill before I went to bed and fell asleep. Awhile later I was awakened by severe stomach pains as though someone had punched me in the stomach. These pains came in waves all night until the desired results occurred. I threw the laxatives in the trash, vowing to never do that again.

Because of my addictive personality that vow was quickly broken. The next night I dug the laxatives out of the trash. I wanted them, had to have them, and continued to take them. I popped another one in my mouth and swallowed. I was going after a different high and thought that since they weren't hard core drugs they were okay to take. The alcohol, bulimia, and the laxatives were just forms of abuse that were meant to cover up my depression and unstable emotions.

All three of my abuses continued in a daily cycle and my health was deteriorating mainly because of the dehydration. One morning I woke up feeling hungover as usual. I grabbed some water and an apple to eat before heading to the beach with some family friends. I spent the entire trip to the beach having moments of dizziness and lightheadedness. I drank some more water hoping that this would improve the situation.

I was in a car with my younger brother and some family friends. They wanted to stop at a fast food place before arriving at the beach. I wouldn't normally eat this kind of food but was so hungry I decided my need to eat overrode my usual nutrition habits. I was so weak that I sat in a chair while waiting to order the food I so desperately needed. I went up to the counter, began to order my food, and began to see stars. I tried to walk back to a chair, dark tunnel vision began, and seconds later I fainted.

I came to consciousness as someone was calling my name. I couldn't understand what happened until my brother told me I had fainted. I slowly sat up and someone brought me some water. As I tried to take a sip of water I fainted again. Another voice brought me back to consciousness. A boy I used to babysit was looking at me with terror in his eyes. My fainting had scared him so he gave me a hug and asked me if I was okay. I said I was fine to keep him from worrying about me.

I glanced over at my brother and saw the shock on his face. I knew that what he had just witnessed must have really scared him. I had a responsibility to be his older sister and his role model but I was failing miserably. I was embarrassed, in shock, and felt like the worst sister in the world. He hugged me and told me that he was glad I was alright noting that he had thought I was going to die. I returned the hug, assured him I was okay, all the while feeling like a complete failure.

The thought of being a failure was something that I didn't handle very well. Instead of doing the right thing and going to the hospital, I shrugged it off as nothing and told everybody that we could go on to the beach. What I didn't understand at the time was that my body was trying to tell me to slow down, nourish properly, and stop drinking. The combination of excessive alcohol consumption and vomiting my food had deprived me of the necessary nutrients and hydration that my body needed. Unfortunately this incident didn't deter me from continuing down a destructive pathway.

I continued drinking whenever I got the chance and didn't miss a chance to attend a party where alcohol was involved. This pattern of behavior began to affect my work ethic and college classes. I started to miss more and more days of school because I was so hungover and exhausted. For the first time I missed a ballet performance because I decided to go out drinking instead. My addiction was ever so slowly surpassing my passion for dance. I was allowing it to slip right through my fingers. I frequently called in to work to say I was too sick to come in when in reality I was just too hungover to get out of bed. I thought this was something every eighteen year old did so didn't think I was doing anything out of the ordinary. I reasoned with myself that at least I wasn't doing illegal drugs or frequently blacking out so I really wasn't doing any harm. The drinking and vomiting continued right through to the end of 2003. Little did I know that 2004 would bring more destruction.

As my nineteenth birthday approached I was filled with anticipation and excitement about being a year closer to moving out of my teen years. My birthday was two weeks away and my friends and parents were already planning special events for me. My dad was going to take me shopping. I was already planning my own night of fun on my actual birthday and wanted to include my best friend. I called her the day before to ask her if she knew of anything going on that night and if she wanted to go out with me. We quickly got a group together, appointed a designated driver which didn't include me, and set out for a night of fun.

We arrived at a friend's house and the drinking began. I decided to drink beer that night instead of hard alcohol so I wouldn't black out and not remember the evening. After about three beers I was pretty buzzed and enjoying the evening. At midnight someone asked me if it was my birthday and I said it was so someone started pouring a round of shots. I had never mixed my alcohol because I had heard that it could be dangerous. Since it was my birthday I took one, then another, and another. I couldn't stop and don't remember how many I had that night. I don't remember leaving the party with my best friend and the designated driver to return to where my car was parked. When we got there my memory started to clear up and I thought about going inside to make plans to spend the night. After that there was some arguing because I suddenly wanted to go home so I could go shopping with my dad in the morning. Someone tried to stop me from driving but I assured them I was fine and drove off toward home.

As I was pulling onto my street I received a birthday text from a friend. She invited me to come out to Hollywood to celebrate. Without thinking I agreed, turned around, and headed toward Los Angeles. I don't remember much about the drive except that at one time I noticed that I was going 100 miles an hour. I quickly reined in and slowed down but saw the flashing lights in my rearview mirror. I didn't panic and pulled off onto the nearest exit. It was the first time I had ever been pulled over by the police and I was pretty wasted on top of it all.

My heart began to race as I saw a male police officer walk up to my window. I popped some gum in my mouth and was prepared to try and get out of it. He asked me if I knew why he had pulled me over and I told him it was because I was speeding. He asked for my license and registration. I started digging around to find it and wondering how much a speeding ticket was going to be. As I handed over the requested items he asked if I had been drinking. I decided that honesty was the best policy so replied that I had had a few beers at a party and was heading to a friend's house in Hollywood.

As he looked at my license he realized that it was my birthday so offered to leave my car there and drive me safely to my friend's house. I was so relieved to hear this and couldn't believe that I had gotten out of a DUI. Up to now I had not been in any serious trouble and wanted to keep it that way. Unfortunately there was a female police officer in the car and she insisted that I come out of the car and take a sobriety test. As I opened the door to my car I knew then and there that I was heading for trouble and that my life would be forever changed. I failed every part of the sobriety test and even fell over attempting to walk a straight line. I tried to blame it on my high- heeled boots but then I heard the words, "Rochelle, you are under arrest..." and I was read my rights.
My entire vision became blurry and I almost fainted. I couldn't

breathe, my heart was racing, and tears began streaming down my face. I felt as though I was in a dream but was snapped back to reality when the handcuffs were placed on my wrists. I began to see flashbacks of myself as a happy-go-lucky child, performing and dancing on stage, and all the other achievements from the past. I realized that those things didn't matter and that what mattered now was that I was being arrested for drinking and driving.

As we drove to the jail my mind was swirling with thoughts and questions. How did this happen to me? Why did I get caught the first time I drank and drove? I was a good kid and never got in trouble. Was I going to jail? What would my parents think about it when they found out? How could I tell my friends? Would they be angry at me? People would probably think I was a troublemaker. I couldn't stop these thoughts and just wanted the nightmare to be over and wake up at home, in my bed, and sober.

The nightmare became a reality when I walked into the police station to begin the booking process. I answered numerous questions, was fingerprinted, and had my picture taken. It felt like my life was going to end as they walked me down a hall and into a cell they called the "drunk tank." Thankfully nobody else was in there so I just curled up in a ball on the floor and waited.

The swirling thoughts from earlier came back with a vengeance. I couldn't stop them from repeating and nagging at my mind. I worried about the disappointment from my parents. I replayed numerous scenarios about how to tell them. A police officer approached my cell and I hoped she was coming to release me but instead instructed me that I was allowed one phone call. She unlocked the door and I rushed over to the phone, dialed my parent's landline, and with a racing heart waited to break the bad news. My mom answered the phone and I blurted out that I was in jail because of a DUI. My mom handed the phone to my dad, I told him what happened, and asked him to come get me out of jail. He said he would do his best and hung up.

The wait felt like two days but in reality was only about six hours. I was completely sober but terribly hungover. I heard my name, stood up, and was told that my dad had posted bail and was there to pick me up. Although I was happy to be released, I didn't look forward to facing my dad. I had always wanted to make him proud and now I was sure this would devastate him. I signed my release papers, took a deep breath, and prepared to greet my dad. As expected, his face showed complete shock and disappointment. He said, "Happy birthday," and we walked to the car in complete silence.

I felt so ashamed that I kept my head down and just wanted to crawl into a hole and never come out. On the way home my dad told me that this wasn't a situation that he ever expected and was a "nice" present I gave myself for my birthday. I said I didn't know what I was thinking, was sorry, and just wanted to go home. He kept driving and told me that he still loved me. His words were a soothing balm on what I considered the worst day of my life.

I walked into my house feeling hungover, dirty, and exhausted. I wanted to take a shower, forget what had happened and celebrate my nineteenth birthday. I walked into my bedroom, took a deep breath, and broke into great heaving sobs which continued through-out my shower. I crawled into bed, looked at my phone for the first time since last night, and saw numerous texts and missed calls. With a heavy heart I dialed my best friend's number and told her what had happened and that it wasn't her fault because she had tried to keep me from driving. She said that she was glad I was still alive, assured me I would get through it, and that she would be there for me. I hung up the phone and began to cry because I knew I had an amazing and loyal friend.

The swirling thoughts from the night before returned and I wondered how I was going to get through this horror! I never once considered that I had a drinking problem. I looked at it as if I had just made a big mistake and I was going to have to deal with the consequences. I asked aloud, "Why me," as if I were the victim. This is a typical response for an addict also known as playing the blame game. I wondered why someone hadn't tried harder to stop me from driving, for example. Then I switched to a pity party of woe is me, or I'm the worst person ever, or I'll never get through this. I just wanted it all to stop and go away.

I heard a knock on my door and knew it would be my mom. I told her to come in even though I was embarrassed by what I had done. She came in, sat down beside me, looked me in the eye and told me that I was going to get through it all and that both she and my father would be there for me. I hugged her and told her how sorry I was. As we were hugging my father came in and said he still wanted to take me birthday shopping and discuss what happened. I agreed and told both of them that I loved them too.

A few weeks passed and I hadn't made any behavior changes. I continued to drink whenever I had the chance to go out and party. I told myself that I was only nineteen and had just made a terrible mistake. I assured myself that I would get over the DUI arrest and all the consequences I would have to endure. Besides, the drinking helped me forget about it all and pretend that everything was alright. I continued attending dance auditions during this time whether I was hungover or not. My aspirations of becoming a super-star performer like Britney Spears had not diminished and this little bump in the road would not keep me from achieving my dream.

I received a call from my agent about a dance audition for an up-coming singer named Jojo. I still had my license and didn't want to miss this opportunity. I drove to Hollywood telling myself that this was just what I needed to distract me from the past few weeks. I walked into the audition and began freestyling for the casting team. In that moment all worries ceased and I was lost in my world of dance performance. I felt powerful and comfortable. I gave them my signature wink at the end of the performance and confidently exited the room. I knew I had given my best performance and had most likely gotten the job. My agent called me as I was driving home and told me that I was booked in the dance video as a featured dancer. I believed that my luck was about to change and my career would be taking off.

Being on the set for my first music video was the experience of a lifetime. Getting my hair and makeup done was secondary to the thrill of being in front of the camera doing what I loved. It was what I lived for and wanted to do for the rest of my life. The video was a hit on Total Request Live which featured popular music videos of the day. I began getting phone calls and texts from people I knew telling me that they had seen me on television. My dream was coming true at last and I was euphoric. It gave me an excuse to go out and celebrate. I didn't really need an excuse to party, but as an addict I rationalized drinking this way.

As I basked in the glow of the music video success, my court date arrived. I had never been inside of a courtroom so didn't know what to expect. I asked my dad to go with me and he agreed. We were ushered into a small courtroom and waited hours for my name to be called. I had no clue what was going to happen so wasn't really that nervous. I tried to maintain good composure and keep my emotions in check. I finally heard my name and was instructed to take the stand.

That's when the terror settled in and my heart began racing. The judge read the details of my case and it all became a terrible reality. I was convicted of driving under the influence, having a blood alcohol level of .19, and driving 100 miles per hour. These three things combined made my case much worse than just a routine DUI. I anxiously awaited to hear my punishment.

The judge admonished me by saying that my case was pretty serious. He mentioned that I could have killed someone else or myself and that my blood alcohol level was over twice the legal limit. I was given the standard DUI fee, alcohol classes, volunteer work, a suspended license for a year, and ninety days in jail! Those last words filled me with fear and I knew that I couldn't spend any time in jail. I thanked the judge and walked back to my father.

I told my dad that there was no way I could do jail time. I had visions in my mind of what prison looked like and none of them were pretty. I feared for my physical safety as well. I expressed these feelings to my dad and he said we would get a lawyer and see what could be done.

We hired a lawyer and at my next court appearance I was sentenced to ninety days in jail or 30 days house arrest. This would mean that I would have a tracking device on my ankle that would monitor my whereabouts and thus keep me in my parent's house. I wouldn't be allowed to leave for any reason. That decision was a no brainer for me. My lawyer set up the court date to get me processed which still meant I had to go to jail for one day. My heart sunk and I felt like I was going to be sick to my stomach. I thought about it for a few days. My lawyer told me that the sooner I turned myself in the quicker it would be over. My court date was set for the next week.

The day quickly approached and as I rolled out of bed I told myself that I just had to get through this day. I got dressed and my dad drove me to the Los Angeles courthouse. I spent the entire drive there telling myself that I was strong and to keep my head held high. It would be one day of hell and then it would be all over.

When my case was called I walked to the stand and it was stated that I was there to turn myself in to be processed for my thirty days of house arrest. As I agreed I looked over at my dad and saw fear and disappointment on his face. I had told my mom to stay home because I was certain that she wouldn't be able to see me walk into a jail. I couldn't imagine what she was going through while at work and thinking about her only daughter going to prison. I mouthed, "I love you," to my dad and was led out of the courtroom.

I was taken to the first processing room, asked to remove my shoelaces and jacket, and any body piercings that could be used as a weapon. I was then walked to the women's side of the jail to be fingerprinted and photographed. I sat on a bench and looked at the women around me. It was like a scene from a movie. I saw prostitutes, criminals, and some obviously mentally unstable women. The woman next to me kept talking to herself and screaming. I tried to assure myself that in a few hours it would be over and I could get out of there.

I was then placed in a holding cell with about ten other women. I found a corner and curled up into a tiny ball to be as far away from the others as possible. A larger woman began approaching me and I thought she was going to physically harm me like I had seen in the movies. Instead I heard her ask me in a soft voice my reason for being there. I told her my story and she asked if she could touch my hair extensions. I felt relieved to know that I wasn't going to be physically harmed.

After what seemed like days but in reality was only a few hours, a policewoman told us to get ready to be moved to another tower. I was handed ugly orange jail clothing with "jail" on the back. I truly felt like a convict at this point. I stood in line with the others, was hand and ankle cuffed, and slowly shuffled toward a bus. I was surprised to see men on the bus so I sat as far away from them as possible, kept my head down, and kept silent.

During the drive I kept thinking about how I just wanted this night-mare to be over. When we arrived and exited the bus, they uncuffed us. I was placed in a room with about fifty women. There was a room next to us that had men in it. There was trash everywhere and the smell was disgusting. I didn't want to talk to anyone so I curled up in a corner again.

After about an hour I was moved into a small cell that was on the women's side of the jail. I felt much safer away from the men so I felt a sense of relief. There were about five other women with me. One girl walked up to me and asked me why I was there. I told her and she told me that she was there because she got caught soliciting sex as a prostitute. Inwardly I cringed and realized that this was not a television movie but my reality. I was thankful for the nice way this girl treated me and I felt a little more comfortable.

The hours slowly clicked by. A female police officer opened our cell and announced that it was time for cavity checks and I wondered what she meant by that. I was shocked when we were asked to strip naked. I was disgusted and embarrassed as I stood there with about twenty other naked women. After the body inspection we had to walk over and take a cold shower. I took the fastest shower of my life and grabbed my prison clothes even quicker. I dressed and was placed in a cell for the rest of the night.

I didn't get any sleep that night. I could hear women talking about sticking needles in their necks, stealing cars, and other violent crimes. I thought about my family and friends and how I just wanted this whole nightmare to be over. Early the next morning I was taken into a very large room with about one hundred beds and numerous tables. I was literally in the heart of the prison. This was where all the women ate, slept, and spent their day. I had to eat disgusting food, brush my teeth with a fake toothbrush and wear the jail uniform. As I sat down on a bench I heard my name called on a loudspeaker announcing that I had a visitor.

I was escorted to a chair that was behind a glass window. I saw my mom walk over, sit down, and pick up the phone. At that moment I knew the gravity of what I had done. My mom had to see me in my prison garb and talk to me on a phone through a plate glass window. I asked her if she knew when I was getting released and she told me they were doing everything possible to make it happen sooner than later.

As she walked away I felt like the biggest failure in the world. The officer took me by the arm and led me back to the jail room. I was beyond exhausted and could barely keep my eyes open so I tried to get a little sleep. I immediately heard my name, got up, and was taken to another, smaller cell with four other women. I was allowed to get dressed in my own clothing. I was hopeful that I would be released soon.

One of the women asked me why I was there and told her about my DUI and impending house arrest. She told me that my time served the past twenty-four hours would serve as my ninety days and that I wouldn't have to do house arrest. I couldn't believe what I was hearing. I was going home and wouldn't have to do house arrest. It sounded too good to be true!

My name was called and I was taken to the check-out area. My clothing and personal belongings were returned to me and I dressed quickly. I was told I could call someone to come pick me up so I called my dad. I had been in the jail for almost two days but it felt like a lifetime. I never wanted to set foot in a jail again. I never considered the real reason that I was there – that I had a problem with alcohol. I just thought I had made a really bad mistake and that after my release things would get better. I promised myself that day that I would never go back to that horrible place.

After I returned home and back to my normal routine, I felt like the worst was behind me. Since I didn't associate my drinking with the reason I had gotten into trouble, I resumed my former partying habits. I still went to school, exercised at the gym, and drank some weeknights. I still drank every weekend but wasn't blacking out so falsely believed that my drinking had improved since my DUI. I still thought I was in a "phase" that would eventually pass. I didn't realize that my alcoholism was lying dormant at this time waiting for the right time to emerge again and eat me alive.

Once I had served my brief prison sentence, my license was suspended for one year. I had to be driven to school, work, or the gym by my parents and friends. I felt like I was fifteen again and extremely embarrassed by it. After thinking about it awhile I came to what I thought was a genius conclusion. Since I wasn't driving I didn't have to worry about getting another DUI so I could drink as much as I wanted. What started out as a punishment turned into an alcoholics dream come true.

My life became more out of control that year. I was drinking during the week, on weekends, and blacking out almost every time. One night I was at a party where everybody was taking hard alcohol shots. I quickly joined in and with the first shot all my problems from the past few months involving my DUI faded away. I was carefree and wanted to keep feeling that way so I took another shot. I was really feeling the effects of the alcohol, having a great time with my friends, so I took another shot. I was in a drunken state at this point but something inside my brain encouraged me to drink more so I took at least three more shots. Some time that night I blacked out and when I woke up awhile later I was inside my friend's car outside her house. I was passed out and my dead weight was too much for her mother and her to handle. I couldn't remember how I had gotten there. I called my friend and asked if I could come inside to sleep and recover. She gave me some water and ibuprofen to help with the eventual hangover. I thanked her and immediately fell asleep.

I woke the next morning feeling like I had been hit over the head with a baseball bat. My head was pounding, my heart was racing and I felt lightheaded. I ran into the bathroom and vomited. The room was spinning out of control so I threw myself onto the floor. I had never felt like this before. What was happening to me? Suddenly the depression hit me and I didn't want to move, think, or eat. My friend knocked on the door and asked if I was alright and offered to drive me home.

As we drove to my house we talked about the night before. Since I couldn't remember what happened after I blacked out, my friend told me how I was talking and not making any sense. I opened up and told her about my depression. She told me that she could relate to my feeling and that maybe I should see a doctor. That idea had never crossed my mind but sounded like a good idea. The problem was that I was an alcoholic and didn't want to have to admit my faults to a stranger so just brushed it off.

Later that day I was lying in bed thinking about how to make my situation better. I never considered that changing my drinking habits would improve things. I thought about how I enjoyed getting ready for dance recitals and putting on makeup. I thought that maybe taking classes to be a makeup artist would be my ticket to feeling better about myself. I could do what I enjoyed and get paid for it. I discussed this with my parents and they agreed to help financially with my new direction. I researched and found a highly recommended school about forty minutes from home. I could take the train since I couldn't drive. I felt excited to be starting something new that was directly related to my future career in the performance industry.

I registered for the course and went to classes five times a week for five weeks. I had my own station with an entire supply of makeup. I enjoyed every moment of the course because I was away from everyone I knew. I didn't drive so I could be hungover and it didn't matter. I could throw up before school started and no one would know. It was an escape from my usual surroundings. My bulimia worsened as I became more obsessed with losing weight to become that "perfect" person I felt I needed to be. I was putting so much pressure on myself that my breaking point seemed inevitable.

The breaking point did arrive and I remember that day like it was yesterday. It started like any other day with taking the train to class, vomiting before class and barely eating the entire day. On this day we were putting on makeup on each other and sitting in front of a real camera on set to see how it projected on screen. When it was my turn all eyes were on me as the teacher discussed my makeup. Another student told me that I looked like a popular actress, Jennifer Aniston, and should be in front of the camera instead of behind it. I thought about it and agreed with her. I didn't want to be behind the scenes putting makeup on the talent but wanted to be the talent.

As others made comments on my makeup my heart began racing, I began to feel hot and started to sweat. The floor began to spin and the walls started to close in around me. I decided that I was having a heart attack from the bulimia habits. I asked to be excused and ran outside. I felt like I couldn't breathe so I hunched over to try and catch my breath. My teacher came out to check on me and I told her this had never happened before. She brought me a snack and water. I began crying and asked if I could call my mom. When I did I told my mom all that was happening. She told me that I had just had a panic attack because she had experienced the same thing years earlier. I was extremely relieved to hear this because it meant that it wasn't my heart. I told her I wanted to come home and go see a doctor.

The panic attack was a clear sign to me that I was having problems. Someone without an addiction would look to the source of the problem, which for me was the drinking, and take care of it in an orderly fashion. Since I was an addict I attributed my current situation to a health problem so I needed to see a doctor. The panic attack had shaken me to the core and I wanted to find a medical reason behind my problems.

I went to the doctor but only told him part of what was happening to me. I told him about my DUI, jail sentence, license suspension and recent panic attack. I didn't tell him about my drinking and bulimia.

He diagnosed me with post-traumatic stress disorder (PTSD) which happens when someone experiences a severely traumatic emotional situation. I'm sure the doctor suspected that I had some type of alcohol issue because when he prescribed some anti-depressants he told me not to drink any alcohol while taking them. I told him I understood his instructions while secretly thinking that I would not follow them.

The medication did nothing but make me sick to my stomach and completely exhausted. I switched to other medications until I found one that didn't make me feel like I had the flu. I still felt like I was drowning and that my life was spiraling out of control. I continued to drink but still couldn't see that this was the root of my problems. I continued to blame those around me for my problems and didn't take responsibility for my actions. I made excuses for everything that was wrong in my life and felt like there was no way out of the hole I was in.

I made no lifestyle changes as I continued to be driven to work and back home, and then go out at night again. My bulimia increased from once a day to up to four times a day. It was the one thing in my life that I could control. I could vomit on demand and it became harder to hide it from my family. I ran water in the bathroom to hide the sound. I took two showers a day so I could vomit in there. I vomited in cups, hid them in the closet, and flushed them late at night to minimize the frequency of toilet flushing. The bulimia actually made me feel better and I felt more powerful, confident, and happy. The drinking also had the same effect. They were my best friends and I never wanted to give them up.

Chapter 5
Hitting Rock Bottom

Hitting rock bottom means that an addict has an event or time in their life when they've reached the absolute lowest point in their disease. This point varies from person to person and is handled in different ways. Faults need to be acknowledged and there needs to be a willingness to change. I was slowly heading in this direction and would have to hit rock bottom before I was able to begin to conquer my alcoholism and eating disorder.

Once I reached the legal age for drinking and had my license reinstated, getting alcohol became much easier. I continued taking anti-depressants, drinking heavily, and having bulimic binges. Blacking out became a regular occurrence. On my twenty-first birthday I drove to the liquor store and bought a bottle of rum. I wasn't celebrating a significant birthday - I believed drinking would fix how I felt. Even though I had a boyfriend, wonderful family and friends, and schooling, I still felt lost. Alcohol was the one thing in my life I could rely on to make me feel happy and powerful.

After I completed makeup school I discovered that booking jobs wasn't as easy as I had anticipated. My mom suggested getting into skincare by going to esthetician school. I agreed it might be something I could be interested in pursuing. I registered for classes and was excited to pursue a new career path. With this new outlook on life I went a few months without drinking one sip of alcohol to prove to myself I could do it. This bolstered my feelings that I truly didn't have a problem with alcohol. The temporary good feelings were still not enough to make me happy or be able to control my drinking for very long.

Esthetician school was forty hours a week, Tuesday through Saturday. This limited my drinking to Saturday and Sunday nights and became "binge" drinking nights. I fully believed I wasn't an alcoholic because I had it in my head that an alcoholic had to drink every day and since I was able to limit mine to just two days, then there was no way I was an alcoholic. Saturday nights became my favorite night of the week because that's when my drinking could begin. My boyfriend became my designated driver. Because he smoked marijuana I rationalized that it was safer for him to drive. My addict brain seriously thought this was true even though driving under the influence of any mind altering substance is unsafe!

As soon as my boyfriend got off work on Saturday nights, we went straight to the grocery store to purchase Bacardi Silver rum which became our go to bottle for Saturday night drinking. We arrived at the party, whipped out my own personal shot glass that I carried in my purse, and immediately began taking shots of the rum. While the other party attendees, mostly my boyfriend's friends, played video games, I drank. I rationalized that since I didn't want to play the games and was bored, the drinking made it more bearable. At the end of the night we went back to my boyfriend's house to spend the night, which wasn't allowed, so I had to sneak in. Rules meant nothing to me if they prevented me from doing what I wanted to do.

Once we got to his house, we sat in his room, continued taking shots, and watched movies until the bottle was empty. I eventually blacked out just before going to bed, remembering everything up to that point and then nothing after. I spent most of the evenings buzzed and then blacked out at the end of the evening having consumed eight to twelve shots. At 5'2" and 112 pounds, that was a very large amount of alcohol.

The morning after hangovers were very intense. When I woke up Sunday mornings I was unable to move at times, my head pounded terribly, and my thirst for water was fierce. Once I was able to get up I grabbed some water, went to the restroom, looked at my reflection in the mirror and asked myself what I was doing to myself. I looked horrible, felt extreme nausea, and I couldn't see a bright future for me beyond this drinking lifestyle I had created. One time I actually felt like punching the mirror in frustration because I wanted the hungover feeling to end.

I tried to freshen up by brushing my teeth but all I could taste while brushing was the rum I had consumed on the previous night. It seemed as if the alcohol was literally coming out of my insides and into my mouth and I had to try and keep from gagging. After brushing I contemplated another way to make myself feel better and remembered the saying, "hair of the dog." This is a colloquial expression that is short for "hair of the dog that bit you" and means to consume a small amount of alcohol to cure a hangover. Since my boyfriend was still asleep, I looked for the bottle of rum we drank from the previous night. I found it and discovered that there was one shot glassful remaining. I measured it out, brought it to my mouth, gagged at the odor, plugged my nose, closed my eyes, and swallowed it. I felt instant relief and was relieved that I had found a new way to cure my hangovers.

I sneaked out of my boyfriend's house, went home, and showered so my parents couldn't smell the alcohol. I dressed and headed back to my boyfriend's to hang out until he went to work. My "hair of the dog" shot from that morning had worn off and a battle was waged between my sensible brain and my alcoholic brain. My alcoholic brain kept telling me to go get more alcohol while my sensible brain said not to. I eventually put my hands over my ears, screamed, and heeded the addict's advice and drove to the store and bought a bottle of rum. I parked down the street from my boyfriend's house and took a swig from the bottle so he wouldn't know I was drinking during the day. I felt instant relief and the voices in my head were silenced.

This pattern of behavior continued as the weeks went by. This vicious cycle was slowly bringing me closer to my rock bottom. I still rationalized that I was no different from any other twenty-one year old who liked to party every weekend with alcohol. I was just having fun.

With the onset of binge drinking my obsession with my weight increased. I started using my bulimia as the reason that I got so drunk. I told my boyfriend that because I vomited my food, I was always drinking on an empty stomach and the alcohol hit faster and harder. I was also, in a way, trying to get help for my eating disorder. My vomiting started to happen involuntarily and I started to lose control over it. The drinking, vomiting, and laxative use needed to be planned out ahead of time so that I could still hide it from others.

The remainder of that year was spent going to school, binge drinking, vomiting, using laxatives, and spending time with my boyfriend. Some days I felt completely in control while other days I felt like I was losing it. For two months I'd have my drinking under control and then the next month I'd lose all self-control. Things would go from being great to feeling like I was in hell. I still didn't want change so I continued with my destructive behavior pattern.

The year came to an end and my twenty-second birthday quickly approached. It had been months since something bad had happened to me, I was vomiting less, and I had graduated from esthetician school. I decided on New Year's to start off the year with a clean slate and made a resolution to not black out while drinking. My goal for drinking had always been to have fun while keeping things under control. I had never wanted to be the "drunk girl" at a party but unfortunately it never ended up that way. Once I started drinking, I literally couldn't stop. My brain craved more and more alcohol until I couldn't control my intake. My resolution to stop blacking out quickly went out the door and became a regular part of my drinking pattern.

After my twenty-second birthday I was at a party for a friend's young daughter. Most of the adults in attendance were drinking but I wanted to wait until everybody had left. Someone offered me a beer and my resolve disappeared. I drank one beer after another, took a break for a few hours until the party ended, and began taking shots of alcohol, eating pizza, and laughing a lot. My friend offered to let me sleep over but I declined and said I was okay to drive home.

With little resistance from my friend, I left the party. I barely remember putting my keys into the ignition and starting my car. As I was driving my phone rang, I reached over to answer it and hit a parked car just down the street from home. I immediately wondered if I should just leave the scene but knew a hit-and-run would be really bad news. As I leaned over to find a piece of paper to write on, I heard a knock on the window. I looked up and my heart sank into my stomach because it was a police officer.

At that moment I knew I was in deep, deep trouble. My mind cleared and I almost felt sober. I was terrified of what I knew was looming in my future. The officer asked me what I was doing and asked for my license after I gave him my explanation. He took my license, walked away, and I knew my previous DUI would show up. When he came back he told me that someone had called 911 and an ambulance was on the way. I told him I was okay and didn't need an ambulance. We chatted while waiting for the ambulance to arrive but I tripped over my own feet and he asked if I had been drinking. I knew it was futile to deny it so I told him I had. I knew then I was going to be arrested again.

I failed the sobriety test and my blood alcohol level was .20 which was 2.5 times over the legal limit of .08. At that moment my dad arrived on the scene, looked at the officer, and told him to take me away. My heart was broken because I had once again disappointed my father and realized that he was letting me face the conse-quences of my actions that night. I began sobbing as I was placed into the back seat of the squad car. As we drove away I began asking myself why this was happening again instead of taking into account that I needed to stop drinking. How could I be so unlucky and why was everybody out to get me?

The more I thought about the situation the more anxious I got. My heart began racing, I overheated, my breaths came in short gasps, and I began having a panic attack. I tapped on the window separat-ing the back seat from the front and told the officer that I couldn't breathe. I was taken to the emergency room of the nearest hospital and given a full check-up while handcuffed to a wheelchair. As the nurse left my room, I mumbled to myself that I wanted to die and that my parents probably would hate me forever. The officer was near enough to hear me and told me that parents loved their kids and wouldn't want them to commit suicide, and that there were a lot worse things in life than what I was going through. His words fell on deaf ears because I just wanted it to all be over.

I was taken to the police station, booked, and placed in the drunk tank. I felt nauseous, light-headed, and extremely tired. I made phone calls to my family and boyfriend, and they all assured me I would get through this terrible situation. I waited six hours for my mom to come pick me up. When she arrived I was so embarrassed I couldn't look her in the eye. I told her I didn't know what was happening to me and I just wanted to go home. I knew she was disappointed, cried all the way home, and felt like I was the worst person ever.

As an overachiever I had always wanted to impress my parents. I not only felt like a weak individual, but that I was a total failure in life. I knew I had talent and was a hard worker but had just thrown it all away with one bad decision to drive while intoxicated. I knew a second DUI conviction would come with more severe consequences and worried I wouldn't be able to live through it. I never once considered if I stopped drinking it would solve all my problems. I blamed it on having bad luck and getting caught. I had gotten myself into this mess and I was going to have to get through it by myself.

My nervousness during my first court appearance was nothing compared to the angst I was feeling at having to face a judge a second time. My DUI had occurred in Ventura County and I had heard that the punishments would be harsher. As I sat in court awaiting my turn, my palms sweated, my heart raced, and my feet shifted nervously.

My name was called and I listened anxiously as the judge read my offenses. He ordered me to take eighteen months of alcohol classes, suspended my license for a year, ordered a breathalyzer for when my license was reinstated, gave me five years' probation, and jail time. I could only respond in the affirmative as I dreaded the nightmare before me.

As I walked out of the courtroom I knew I could handle all the punishments except the jail time. The two days I had spent previously were shear torture and I knew I wouldn't be able to handle a longer sentence. I discussed this with my lawyer and he suggested doing a work furlough program. I could either serve about ten percent of my jail sentence at no cost or join the work furlough program for the full thirty days with a large monetary cost. I would have to spend the night at the facility and work five days at my regular job. My parents agreed that jail was not a place they wanted me to be and offered to pay for my entry into the work furlough program. I knew the program wouldn't be easy but a much better option than the unsafe environment of jail time.

I already had a job at a salon near home as an esthetician. I was required to inform my employer about being enrolled in the program. This meant that I wouldn't be allowed to leave work for any reason and someone from the program would randomly drop in to make sure I was there. I could also be given random breathalyzer tests. My employer was required to sign off that she was willing to have me work under these conditions. I was humiliated but thankful I wasn't going to have to serve jail time and she agreed to the conditions of the program. I was now ready to begin serving my thirty-day sentence.

My mom drove me to the work furlough building to get me checked in. I began crying out of fear because I didn't know what to expect on the inside. She reminded me that this choice was a far better one than jail time and I had to agree. I held my head high and walked into the building. I got a room with three other women and thought that it looked just like a jail cell with colors. The food, housing, and bathrooms were awful. There was quite the variety of women in residence and my first overnight was beyond hell to me. I cried softly when I went to bed and didn't sleep all night because my roommate was loudly snoring. The loss of bathroom privacy kept me from being able to vomit after eating. I also would not be able to drink or do physical exercise the entire stay. All my favorite things had been taken away but I blamed only myself. I still never entertained the possibility I had a problem with alcohol and it was the root of all my trouble.

One night as I was sitting in my bunk I saw one of my roommates reading a really thick blue book. I asked her what she was reading and she told me it was a book from Alcoholics Anonymous. I had never heard of the book or the organization but quickly told her I wasn't an alcoholic since I was able to stop drinking any time I wanted and the only reasons I was in there were being unlucky and getting caught. She remained silent as I spoke, but I am sure she knew inside I was in denial about my drinking. I just wanted to serve my sentence and go home and back to my drinking and partying. It's all part of the insanity of being an alcoholic.

After two weeks I was bored and decided I missed physical exercise so I began doing abdominal crunches, pushups, weight exercises with water bottles, and running in place. I instantly felt better and my head cleared. I hadn't had any alcohol in two weeks and the exercise improved how I felt and I discovered I could think straight. I didn't know it at the time, but fitness was going to play a major role in the future.

The thirty-day work furlough ended right on time because I was on good behavior. I had put in my time but had not received any good counsel on my drinking problem so when I was released I was the same person who had entered the program a month earlier. I still didn't think I was an alcoholic but rather a woman with bad luck and as I walked out of the building for what I hoped was the last time, I told myself I would never do that again. I would go back to drinking but use great caution.

Since my boyfriend was in Europe on vacation, I made plans with a friend to celebrate not drinking for thirty days by drinking again. That is insanity at its finest. I went right back to my former habits and dug myself into a deeper hole. I ordered a drink and that first sip was amazing and I felt instantly buzzed. The warmth of the alcohol as I swallowed it gave me the false impression of happiness and I loved it.

Since I couldn't drive I didn't have to worry about the amount or frequency of my drinking. I resumed drinking during the week because I wasn't driving myself to work. It became a very scary situation for me. The blackouts increased until I was blacking out every time I drank. It didn't matter what I drank or how much I drank, I blacked out one hundred percent of the time.

My drinking always started out the same way. I would have one or two drinks, feel buzzed, happy, and be having a good time. Then suddenly a switch inside my brain would go on and compel me to drink more and more alcohol. The demon inside me was insatiable and no amount of alcohol seemed enough. I eventually blacked out after only four or five drinks or shots. Sometimes it happened after only one drink. I was still taking Wellbutrin and that combined with alcohol was beyond toxic. I didn't care because I wanted to drink and that was all that mattered.

As my drinking worsened I began losing friends. If someone wanted to give me advice I pushed them away. If someone wanted to drink with me, they became my best friend. To clarify this, I was losing friends who clearly cared about me and my well-being. They loved me and knew the person I was before alcohol took over. They wanted only the best for me and could see I was going down the wrong path. My circle of friends now included those who were already alcoholics or had other destructive issues. I was surrounded by an unhealthy, toxic, and going nowhere crowd. All my former friends who had goals in life wanted nothing to do with me when I was drinking or drunk. I was going nowhere but downhill at this time.

My year's suspension was finally up and I was granted a restricted license with a breathalyzer installed in my car. I had to breathe into it to be able to start my car and every fifteen minutes after that. If the device detected even the smallest amount of alcohol, a report was sent to my probation officer. This restriction would last another year and gave me the freedom to drink as much as I wanted because I couldn't drive my car with any alcohol in my system. This would keep me safe from another DUI.

As my alcoholism worsened, so did my bulimia. It was the one area in my life that I felt I could control. I could control when and how I wanted to do it. I began to research on the internet ways in which to conceal it and different ways to carry it out. I became almost obsessed with it and kept it from everybody except my younger brother. Our bathroom connected and he eventually caught on to my behavior, told my mom, who then confronted me about it. I vehemently denied it and told her he must be mistaken.

After my mom confronted me, I ran to my room, worried about how bad it was getting, and began researching the side effects of bulimia. I discovered it was not only bad for your teeth, stomach and esophagus but could also cause heart attacks. I became extremely scared at the prospect of yellow teeth, esophageal damage or dying of a heart attack so I decided to quit the vomiting right then and there. I literally quit cold turkey and never looked back at that eating disorder, ever! I felt disgusted I had allowed myself to develop such a horrific addiction. As I turned off my computer I vowed to never voluntarily vomit again and felt freedom from ridding myself of this addiction. I never went back to it.

Even though I had won a victory over my eating disorder, I continued drinking. Without the worry of hiding my vomiting I had more time to think about how and when I could drink. The cessation of vomiting was a good thing but the pain and suffering inside of me was still there. If something went wrong I drank. If something went right I drank. I didn't need a reason to drink any longer and could drink whenever I wanted to. Things got so bad my boyfriend had to tell me what happened the previous night. I blacked out every time we drank on the weekend and couldn't remember anything I had done and wondered if I had done something bad, embarrassing, or simply passed out in bed. I awakened in a state of self-pity and loathing and felt like this could possibly be the lowest point in my life. Even though I was unhappy I would not stop drinking.

The continued alcohol abuse slowly eroded my self-confidence and I became extremely unhappy in my relationship with my boyfriend. I needed someone who was able to take care of me, help me get better by going the distance and doing whatever it took to fix or solve my problems. This is a complete turnaround from the fiercely independent young woman I had been just a few years previously. The alcohol addiction made me feel worthless, lacking in talent, and a nobody going nowhere. The hardest part was deep down inside I didn't want to be any of those things. I wanted to be known as a strong individual both mentally and physically.

My boyfriend couldn't handle the woman I wanted to become. I began spending more time with the girlfriends I still had, separating myself from him as often as I could. There was extreme jealousy on both sides and I wanted the space to broaden my horizons and he resented that. I didn't like him spending time with other females who took interest in him. All of this caused a vicious non-stop cycle of conflict between us which almost always took place while we weren't sober.

The jealousy issue became so extreme that I felt trapped. I didn't want to break his heart but needed to get out of the toxic relationship. The conflicts continued along with the good times until we both decided to go our own separate ways. We wanted different things in life and needed to take our own paths in order to do that. I apologized for any hurt I had caused him and wished him the best. He said the same and our relationship came to an end.

I felt like a weight had been lifted off my shoulders and could now move on to a new chapter in my life. My license had been fully restored and the breathalyzer removed. I was still working as an esthetician and living with my parents. I assumed I would be happy as I once was but found instead I was still greatly depressed and turned to alcohol more than before. I could now drink as much as I wanted to without worrying about checking in with a boyfriend. I lived a crazy, insane, out of control lifestyle because I was now free and on my own. I stayed away from home several days a week, wearing the same clothes for days and bringing makeup and a toothbrush in case I didn't go home. This meant that my drinking binges were premeditated. How crazy was that?

As I moved through life I still managed to keep a few of my true girlfriends. One of my best friends invited me to her birthday party on a party bus that went to Hollywood. I didn't have to worry about driving and could stay overnight with her if I didn't feel like going home. I took two shots for the drive down so that I could be completely buzzed before going into the club. I drank heavily, got punched in the face when boarding the bus to come home, and woke up at another girl's house wearing my clothes from the party. I looked in the mirror and was surprised I had no bruising from the altercation.

I called my best friend to find out the details of the fight. She told me it was the other girl's fault but at that point it didn't matter. If I had been sober I wouldn't have gotten punched in the first place because I could have either defended myself or walked away. Nobody knew the exact details but what mattered most was I felt mentally and physically exhausted. I knew I couldn't go on in this manner. I craved for peace, sanity and success, not a life full of drama and insanity.

I knew I needed to make some serious changes in my life and started to think about fitness and exercise because I had always enjoyed being active. I was still blind to the effects that alcohol was having on my life and was grasping at straws in another direction in hopes of fixing what was wrong inside of me.

I began taking bicycle spin classes almost every day and grew to admire and respect two of the women instructors. I felt empowered, happy and sane when I completed a class which is the polar opposite of how alcohol made me feel. It gave me a good kind of high and helped me maintain my slender physique. Both of the instructors were runners and had completed race distances of half and full marathons. I soon found myself wanting to be like these women, both mentally and physically strong.

After several months of taking regular spin classes, one of the instructors approached me and said she had a half marathon training plan for me. She told me she was confident I could follow the plan and do the race distance. I was doubtful since I had never run six miles let alone 13.1. She was totally unaware of my struggle with alcohol or that I was someone who couldn't turn down a challenge. I looked over the training plan when I got home and decided to embark on my first half marathon journey.

I was entering into foreign territory but was willing to try. I thought maybe this would be the solution to my problems. I set a goal to complete every day on the schedule and I stuck to it. I wanted to run that half marathon and feel proud of myself. I hadn't felt that way in years. I had new goals and direction in my life. Everything seemed to be falling into place until I got a phone call the night before the race.

My instructor was letting me know she was at a nearby club. My mind went immediately to drinking mode and all those weeks of training and preparation for the race went right out the window. My instructor had no idea I had a problem with alcohol and probably thought I would join her, have a couple of drinks, go home, and get up for the race the next day. Instead, I woke up at her house the next morning so hungover I was unable to get up, go to the race and run.

I couldn't believe I had put in all that hard work and missed the race because of alcohol. I was terribly disappointed and ended up lying to my parents about the race. I told them I had run the race because if I told them I had missed it they would know the reason. After telling them this lie right to their faces, I went to my room and fell asleep feeling completely ashamed of myself. I realized that fitness wasn't going to be the key to solving my alcohol addiction.

I still thought my drinking was just a phase I was going through and would eventually disappear with time. I still had my job as an esthetician, enjoyed my fitness training and classes, all the while continuing with my binge drinking. It was like riding a roller coaster with ups and downs. I was able to handle my alcohol at times but was completely out of control other times. My emotions went from feeling terrific and happy to horrible and despondent.

In October 2009 I decided to train for another half marathon. I followed the plan to a tee and didn't miss a day of training even though I was still binge drinking. I was determined to not repeat past mistakes and kept myself from drinking the night before the race. When I stepped onto the course, I got a rush similar to a runner's high. The race hadn't started yet but I was certain that I was going to like it.

The race started and I began my half marathon journey. By mile ten

I wanted to quit and began crying. I told myself I would never do it again, I would get through it, and I would keep going. I was tired and out of breath so I walked a little to regain my composure. I persevered and crossed the finish line in two hours and thirteen minutes. I saw my parents there supporting me with a look of joy on their faces. I felt like I had finally made them proud of me and decided I would do this race distance again. When I returned home I registered for my second half marathon eight weeks later.

I followed through on the training for my second half marathon and finished in December 2009. My finish time was two hours and three minutes, ten minutes faster than my previous race. To celebrate I went out drinking with my running friends and spin instructor. We all took some shots and continued into the night. Everybody else had about two or three but that wasn't enough to feed my alcohol addiction. After everyone went back to their hotel rooms, I purchased a small bottle of vodka, went to a public bathroom stall, and started taking swigs from the bottle. I continued this way to quiet the voice in my head that told me I needed more. I couldn't stop for anything or anyone.

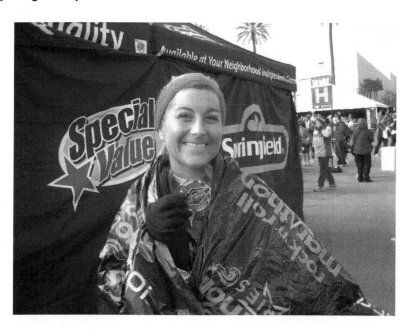

My passion for running and racing continued to grow but my binge drinking didn't decrease. My spin instructor told me I should enter a marathon on January 17, 2010. I was incredulous, told her she had to be kidding, and said there was no way I could complete a race of 26.2 miles. She told me I could do it if I wanted it bad enough. I decided I needed to prove to myself I could conquer a full marathon, and maybe in the process, I could conquer my drinking problem. I started training with the race looming just a mere four weeks away. I vowed not to miss a single day of training in order to perform at my very best.

I broke that promise in a matter of weeks. I was too hungover to do the scheduled twenty mile run and had to call my running friend to tell her I couldn't make the run. I lied and told her I was sick and I would do the run another day. She believed me and told me to get better and do it later that week.

I managed to complete the remainder of my training days while continuing to binge drink. I literally had to make the decision about whether I wanted to run or be hungover the next day and drinking usually won the battle. I got to the starting line, unprepared, but determined to accomplish my goal. At mile nineteen I told myself I needed to own this moment and when I crossed the finish line I could go reward myself. Of course this meant drinking! I crossed the finish line in four hours and forty- four minutes and knew at that moment I loved the sport. I forgot about drinking as my mind experienced the runner's high. I was happy, excited, and very proud of my accomplishment. I knew I would do it again.

When I got back to the hotel, I felt like a new person. I hadn't felt this way since I had won the big dance scholarship. I felt like my former happy and proud self. I could now boast that I had finished my first full marathon on my 25th birthday. I called my parents and told them the good news and I could hear the pride in their voices. After the call ended my addiction began calling my name and I had one beer to celebrate. The switch in my brain to have more alcohol was instantly turned on so I declined an invitation for dinner out, stayed alone and drank until I was tired enough to pass out before my friends returned.

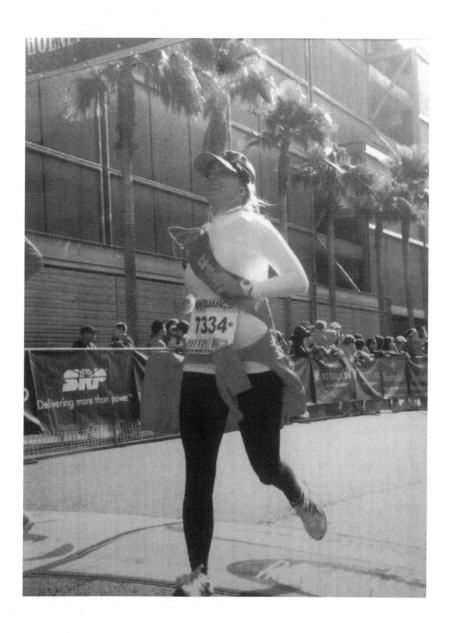

I was slowly coming to the conclusion that running wasn't helping my drinking problem and it was getting worse. I knew deep down using my birthday as an excuse to drink was just another reason to justify my drinking right after a marathon. It was at this point in time I admitted to myself I was an alcoholic. I drank when I was happy, sad, angry, jealous, or excited. It didn't matter how I was feeling, I just had to drink. My alcoholism had completely consumed me.

Although I admitted to myself that I was an alcoholic, I didn't want to admit it to my family and friends. I was embarrassed and felt like a failure. I was going to have to hide it and continue running marathons as a cover up. I completed another full marathon six weeks after my first one. I still missed numerous days of training and had a stress fracture in my foot. This second marathon was miserable due to the pain in my foot and the ongoing battle in my mind about whether I wanted to continue through life as a drinker or a runner. My addiction was still winning at this point. My body craved the alcohol and demanded more and more.

I continued drinking and lying about it, and disappearing for days to keep my parents from seeing me drunk. I stayed with friends and would binge drink for two to three days in a row. Eventually it became obvious to those around me because I sent texts when drunk that gave away my drunkenness. Family and friends knew what was happening but didn't know what to do to help me. I was sinking into a black hole and felt completely lost. My sober brain still wanted me to be successful in life, but my addiction quickly squashed this thinking and kept gnawing at me until I gave in and drank again. I had never been a quitter but was losing the battle quickly.

My parents and friends who truly cared about me became so concerned that they suggested Alcoholics Anonymous (AA) meetings. I didn't think that was the solution to my problem but went to one meeting just to get my parents off my back. I hated every moment of the meeting, thought it was ridiculous, and couldn't publicly admit I was an alcoholic. I told my parents I wasn't going back. My depression returned and getting out of bed, exercising, and socializing became difficult. I rationalized the only thing that brought me happiness was alcohol. Nothing mattered in my world but drinking and I began drinking alone.

I knew I was letting everybody down including myself. I felt hopeless and unable to dig myself out of the deep, dark hole I was in. In desperation I decided that I needed a cry for help and swallowed eight Wellbutrin washed down with alcohol. I didn't really want to die so as soon as things started to get fuzzy and I felt dizzy, I told my parents. They rushed me to the hospital emergency room and while we waited my mom told me that if I died she would be both sad and mad at me. She said she didn't want to lose her only daughter. This was a defining moment for me because I knew that in spite of all I had done and put her through, she still loved me. My dad, on the other hand, couldn't even look me in the eye because the thought of losing me was unbearable. He took a picture of how I looked lying in the hospital bed: wearing a robe, smeared makeup all over my face, and drinking charcoal to absorb the medication I had ingested. Then he told me he wanted his beautiful, talented, successful daughter back.

He was right. I had become a completely different person from the alcohol addiction. It had taken my life away from me. Everything that was important to me was gone. The addiction overshadowed these thoughts and I left the hospital unchanged. I was unwilling to make the necessary changes. I just wanted the alcoholism to disappear and continue to drink like someone without an addiction.

The hospital scare wasn't enough to make me change my drinking habits. I continued binge drinking on the weekends. During one of these binges I reconnected with a former high school friend. I went to school with his aunt who was a good friend of mine. I knew he had been involved in drugs and alcohol and had changed from the sweet, handsome, success-bound guy I used to know. I thought catching up with him was a good idea because I could tell he liked to drink.

I had no intention of getting into any kind of relationship with him because I was too far into my alcoholism to bother with such a thing. There was one pivotal night when I realized that he was just like me. He told me all about how he used hard core drugs but stopped using them. He talked about wanting to get into the Navy and about his personal struggles. He had turned to drugs and alcohol when everything seemed to be going for him and his future, which matched my life's journey. I felt as though our similarities caused us to understand each other and I became head over heels in love with him.

As I spent more time with my new boyfriend, I saw how deeply he was into his own alcoholism. His mother was extremely lenient in allowing us to drink at her house which made it the perfect place for me to spend much of my time. I only returned to my parents' home to get clothes and personal items I needed. The freedom to drink made my drinking become a daily habit causing me to miss work and eventually get fired from one of my jobs for not showing up as scheduled. After a month of this behavior, my parents gave me the choice to move out or go into a rehabilitation program.

I knew I would not be able to make it on my own since I was working minimal hours and drinking too much. I knew that if I didn't go into rehab I would end up on the streets. So after much thought I checked into a program. When I arrived I observed both men and women who looked like they had just arrived from prison. I was so terrified the first night I started sobbing and wanted to get out of there. I begged my parents to switch me to an outpatient program where I would spend the day at the rehab facility and sleep at my parent's house at night. Being there brought back the nightmares from my two previous jail times.

I was relieved when my parents allowed me to continue with the outpatient program for thirty days. I was able to stay at my parent's house at night and feel safe. Unfortunately I was only going through the motions because in actuality I really didn't want to get better. I was only doing the program to appease those around me, especially my parents. I knew from day one I would go back to drinking and being part of the program just gave the appearance of caring and wanting to get better.

I came out of rehab as a "dry drunk" which means I wasn't drinking at that particular time but hadn't made any internal emotional or behavioral changes. I completed my thirty days in rehab, went without alcohol for five months, and wasn't involved in an Alcoholics

Anonymous (AA) program. I thought AA was nonsense and barely attended meetings. My family and friends were happy I wasn't drinking but I hated every moment of it. The only positive aspect for me was not having a hangover. I was angry I wasn't supposed to drink and cringed inwardly as I watched my boyfriend drink beer when we were together. I missed alcohol, knew what pain and suffering it would bring, yet didn't care.

One night while watching a movie at my boyfriend's house, I got up to get some water from the refrigerator. When I opened the door I saw an open bottle of wine and my addiction starting talking to me telling me to drink the wine. My heart told me not to but I quickly ignored it, grabbed the bottle, and took a swig. I felt the cold wine go down my throat and into my stomach, bringing the instant relief it had always brought. I grabbed a cup, poured some more, and thus ended my five-month sobriety. The next morning I had one of the worst hangovers I had ever experienced. The suffering wasn't physical but instead overwhelming feeling of self-pity, embarrassment, and sadness. I felt like a complete failure because I let my addiction win again.

The guilt I felt from breaking my five-month sobriety was so unbearable I decided to give it another try. I kept my one night of drinking to myself because I didn't want to disappoint anybody. I remained sober for another four months and carried on with my life as if everything was alright. At this time I decided it was time to try and live on my own. As I made this decision I knew in my heart I wasn't going to remain sober because I wouldn't be accountable to anybody but myself. I wouldn't have to lie or hide it from anyone.

The move into my new home went well with my parents helping me. Everything was moved in and I felt free at last. After my parents left, I grabbed my keys and drove to the liquor store down the street. I bought a bottle of vodka and some diet soda to chase it with. I returned home, called my parents to thank them for helping me, and while I was on the phone with them I took my first drink in four months. That's how an addiction takes over. I didn't care about anything at that moment except drinking and I felt happy, excited, amazing, and at peace.

My addiction rapidly worsened and I planned my entire life around drinking. I began with binging on the weekends and progressed to binging during the week. I called in sick to work more than I ever had. I personally called clients to tell them I was sick and had to reschedule their appointments. The hangovers became so intense that I had to take a shot in the morning just to feel better. I failed miserably at hiding my intoxication because my phone calls and text messages were a dead giveaway. I thought I could hide my drinking from my boyfriend when we were together because he was battling his own inner demons.

Mornings and evenings began to blur together and I struggled through each day until I could go home and drink. I binged three or four days non-stop and then would take a few days to sober up and recover. I experienced blackouts every time I drank and have very few memories of my "hitting rock bottom" moments. My life became a black screen where I couldn't see or remember anything. I only know what happened because of the stories related by my true friends, parents, and boyfriend.

The heavy, constant drinking finally got to my boyfriend and he began to lose interest. He told me that he couldn't handle my drinking on top of his own personal battle with addiction. I literally felt like my world came crashing down on me. My parents were furious with me, my true friends were gone, and now I lost someone I truly loved. I still wanted to be with him in spite of his addictions and felt a connection because of that. I was literally on my own without anyone to help me.

At the store I went to pay for my purchase and realized my identification and debit card had been in the bag I threw out the car window. I drove back to where I had discarded the bag and dug around in the bushes until I found my belongings. I drove back to the store, purchased the vodka, and as I pulled into my driveway I sat in my car and thought about what had just happened. I had been on my hands and knees, digging through the bushes to retrieve something I had carelessly thrown out the car window. It was pure insanity and it was my life at the moment.

I unfastened my seatbelt and stared at the vodka bottle I had purchased. My thought swirled about the happy girl I used to be and who was completely gone because of alcohol. I felt hopeless and defeated. I unscrewed the bottle cap and for a second considered putting down the bottle. I told myself that if I did I could get back everything that was important to me and I could become the woman I had always wanted to be. I wanted to be successful and proud of myself but was too weak at the moment. My addiction had completely consumed me and I felt as though I had lost the battle.

I was now at the lowest point in my life. I knew at that point I was a full-blown alcoholic and couldn't stop drinking even though I knew it was the right thing to do. This was how my life was going to be - miserable and consumed by my alcoholism. I took a swig from the bottle, went inside my house, and drank until I blacked out and passed out on my bedroom floor next to a pile of crackers.

The next morning I woke up, still on the floor, hurting all over physically and emotionally. I checked my phone, saw that I had tried to call my former boyfriend over thirty times, but had no memory of this. Several people had texted to check on my well-being. My head was spinning and I felt like I was going to vomit everywhere. I searched for the vodka bottle from the night before and discovered that there was enough remaining for one final swig.

As I brought the bottle to my lips the inner conflict began. My brain told me not to do it while my alcoholism screamed, "Do it!" I was sick and tired of the miserable life I was living and letting alcohol win the battle. I walked outside to get some fresh air still carrying the vodka bottle. I threw the bottle against the fence, shattering it and all it stood for. Alcohol had brought me nothing but pain and suffering for the past six years and I was determined to fight to win the battle raging inside of me.

Chapter 6
Road to Recovery

"There's nothing better than the natural high you get from finishing a marathon or an Ironman. I'd never trade that for a drink." – Rochelle Moncourtois, Ironman Journal entry. 7/29/12

Everything in my drunken world was about to change after I made the tough decision to get sober. There was no doubt in my mind I was completely done with drinking. I was beat up, exhausted, and ready to do anything to overcome this addiction. This would be the first step on my journey to sobriety.

I grabbed my phone and dialed my parents to tell them about my decision to get sober. The sound of relief in their voices was pure joy to me. I think they both knew I was serious and truly ready to change my life. I then called my spin instructor to share my good news because she was my closest friend at the time. She had witnessed my drunkenness, saw me flake on training days, and even tried to help me stop drinking. Her response to my news was to ask me if I wanted to be an alcoholic or an athlete. The answer was a no brainer for me. I was ready to move on to a new chapter in life as a sober athlete.

From that moment on I was extremely serious about my recovery. I checked into a private rehabilitation program which I felt was the right fit for me. This time would be different because I finally admitted I was an alcoholic, wanted to change, and was prepared to leave my current environment to get well. I was ready to move forward with my former goals of success and return to the happy girl I once was. I knew for all this to happen I needed to check into a rehab program and truly get sober.

I knew I needed to be in an inpatient rehab program in order to get well, but was terrified at the prospect. My dad drove me there and my hands were sweaty and shaky. I began crying before I got out of the car, not out of sadness, but relief. I was ready to give up alcohol forever which gave me the confidence that my life was eventually going to change for the better.

The whole premise of rehab is this - all that was familiar and comfortable had to be left behind. That meant no cell phone or internet and no contact with family or friends for thirty days. I knew this separation was totally necessary for my journey to sobriety.

After getting settled in my recovery began. I was taught the proper tools to recover from alcoholism and had access to counselors to talk to about anything on my mind. I attended three Alcoholics Anonymous (AA) meetings a day. This time my eyes, ears, and heart were open to what I heard during the meetings. I stayed quiet and listened to other people's stories about how they got sober. Nobody had a story that matched my own, but I still received great information. I absorbed the information I needed in order to finally be free from alcohol.

One aspect of the program was art therapy. I was asked to cut out magazine clippings to explain my life goals and what I wanted from sobriety. As I read my goals my counselor was extremely impressed with my first one which was to compete in and finish a 140.6 mile Ironman Triathlon. I explained it had been a dream of mine for awhile but hadn't been possible because of my drinking and now I wasn't just going to try to do it, I was going to do it. I wanted to write a book, start a fitness clothing brand, and become a personal trainer on the hit television show: "The Biggest Loser." I explained that I had always been a goal setter and had never quit anything in my life except alcohol. Then I told her, "When you want something bad enough, you will find a way just like I did with drinking. Now I want these goals in life and I want to make a difference and be a good role model."

Later that night, I thought over my afternoon therapy session and decided I very much wanted to change my life. I wanted to motivate and inspire others. I wanted to prove to myself I could do anything I put my mind to. In order to achieve all this, I knew without a doubt, that I needed to complete my rehab program and remain sober. It was going to be a challenge and failure was not an option!

As the first two weeks of rehab passed, I could feel myself getting physically and mentally stronger. My thinking was realistic, peaceful, and sane. It was the first time in six years I truly felt at peace with myself and I was ready to make the next big step. In another session I was asked to write a letter addressed to "alcohol" in which I broke off our relationship. To a "Normie" this might sound trivial, but to an alcoholic it is an extremely hard task. My relationship with alcohol, although tumultuous, was long standing and one that I was used to. The relationship was toxic and I needed to cut it completely out of my life.

"Dear Alcohol, You have brought me nothing but pain and misery for about six years of my life. Sure, we had fun at first getting buzzed and partying it up. There were a lot of fun times, but then it took a turn for the worse. You became poison for me. Every time I drank you, you completely took over me. I lost all control and inhibitions when you were in my system. You turned me into a monster and someone who wasn't truly me. Most of the time you made me blackout, leaving me feeling completely lost. I started to lose not only myself, but my family and friends too. I became dependent on you. I started to use you more and more often. The binges became more frequent and the depression became worse. It became so bad, I even wanted to kill myself over you. You made me lose my confidence, strength, and determination in life. I was losing everything important in my life because of you. You pretty much are the devil and give people a false sense of happiness. You never made me actually happy, you made me feel terrible about myself. For some reason, I would still go back to you every time no matter what happened. I was addicted to you and your toxic ways, until now. Now I am becoming a different person. I no longer want or need to rely on you for anything. After two weeks of being free from you, I have become a hell of a lot stronger. I'm physically getting my strength back and mentally focused. You will NOT control me or my life anymore. You are one tough son of a bitch, but now I'm stronger. This is the day I

get to win the battle and completely break up with you. After all the pain and suffering you put me through, I'm done. You no longer serve a purpose for me and I despise you. Goodbye forever. Sincerely, Rochelle"

Although this letter was one of the hardest to write it was the best letter I had written. I officially became sober that day even though I hadn't had a drink in weeks. My mind was set free and I was rid of a toxic and deadly relationship that was bringing me down. I felt powerful when I read my letter aloud to my counselor at a park near my former high school. I thought about all the happy memories before my alcoholism took root. I was ready to be that happy-go-lucky girl again and it felt as though a huge weight had been lifted off my shoulders. When I finished the reading of my letter I asked my counselor if I could go for a short run in the park.

I ran lap after lap thinking about my new freedom from alcohol. I had no music, just the sound of my footsteps hitting the dirt path. I could see my high school as I was making loops round the park and thought about the goals I had set for myself six years earlier to be a dance performer. I decided maybe that goal was not in my cards and a new direction might be a better choice. I continued running and thought about how my life was going to change for the better by overcoming my addiction to alcohol. I came to a complete stop and came to the sudden realization that I wanted to be an athlete again. I felt strong, confident, and in control. I knew then running was going to be my new passion without the encumbrance of alcohol and its crazy effect on my body and my life.

I decided to keep my epiphany to myself and show others by my actions instead of words. I had already completed several half and full marathons while an alcoholic, so completing an Ironman was surely within my capabilities. The last few days in rehab were more than special to me as I learned all the tools I needed to remain sober. I had groundbreaking moments that would shape by future. My thirty day sobriety chip was held tightly in my hand and I thanked the individuals that had been instrumental in my progress through the program. Tears of joy flowed freely as I stepped out of rehab that day thinking: "I'm free!" I was embarking on a new beginning, free from the debilitating grip of addiction and alcohol.

After leaving rehab I moved back in with my parents and began Alcoholics Anonymous meetings immediately. I needed the security and structure in my personal environment before I felt comfortable living on my own. Stepping back into my childhood room was the hardest part of coming out of rehab. The drunken, morning- after memories came flooding back to me. I could almost smell the alcohol even though the room was completely clean. I threw down my bags, took a deep breath, and reminded myself those days were gone forever and I was presently in a loving, sane environment where I could maintain sobriety.

After getting my belongings in order, I went directly to my computer to follow through on the goal I set while in rehab. I didn't waste any time thinking about it and with one click I was registered for a full Ironman triathlon. I was locked in to conquer my quest at only thirty days sober. I knew the components of this arduous event but didn't care. I was more than mentally ready to work towards a 2.4 mile swim, 112 mile bike ride, and 26.2 mile run.

Even though I was registered for my first full Ironman triathlon, I didn't start training until January 1, 2012. It was the beginning of a new year, I was ninety days sober, and I was ready to begin my Ironman training. I decided to keep a journal of my journey over the next seven months.

Day 1 - January 1, 2012
"Today is my 1st day of base training. I did a 15.6 miler on my bike. I'm still really slow, but I'll get better. I documented my ride on camera. I'm excited, nervous, and a little scared for this journey to start. Let the fun begin!"

I was literally at the bottom with cycling. I rode a few short rides the previous week on a borrowed bike from a friend and wasn't using clip-in pedals yet. I was terrified to brake for the first time because I couldn't remember which leg to set down. I stayed in one gear the entire fifteen miles and wore a pair of running shoes. I felt slow as numerous cyclists passed me and the entire ride lasted what felt like an eternity. The thought of riding the full 112 miles in the race seemed more than daunting. This ride left me so sore I could barely move.

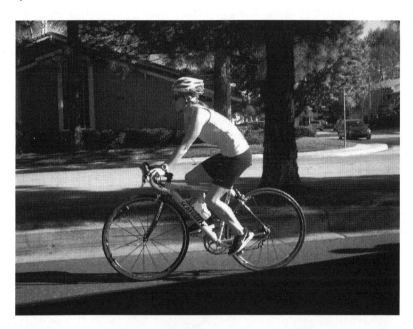

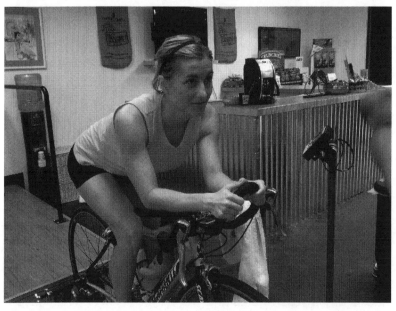

I knew I needed a cycling coach and called one recommended by a friend. I would not conquer the bike overnight and it was going to be an uphill battle for the next seven months. It wasn't going to be easy but I wanted it badly enough to do the hard work. My first day consisted of practicing braking over a hundred times, cycling in circles, and maneuvering around cones. I was totally out of my comfort zone and could see I had a long journey ahead of me.

Day two of Ironman training was a little easier because running was my strongest event so I was most comfortable in that element. Running made me feel strong both mentally and physically. Doing a track interval workout was hard, but I loved it!

Day 2 – January 2, 2012
"Run track workout. 5 miles of sprints: 4x400 @ 7.5, 800 pace, 6x800 @ 7.0, 8:30 pace. I did really well with the workout today."

My training schedule called for a 1,500 meter swim as my first pool workout. That distance is almost half of the 2.4 mile Ironman distance so I would need over 2,300 meters more, in open water, to complete the swim segment of the Ironman. This seemed so far out of reach, but my background in swimming as a child would benefit me now. I remembered my stroke and breathing technique so was able to get through the workout much easier than if I had started from scratch. I was slow but speed wasn't my goal. I wanted to complete it with proper form.

Day 3 – January 3, 2012
"Swim: 200 meters, 20x50 meter sprints, 300 meters. The sprints killed me! Swimming sprints make me want to throw up!"

After three weeks of training I was scheduled to do "bricks" which are workouts that include two or all three of the events in one training day. The purpose is to get used to transitioning from one event to another. The first time I did a cycle/run brick, I felt like my legs had heavy bricks tied to them. I could barely get my legs going and it took almost thirty minutes to get into a good running rhythm.

This new training technique was going to be a whole process.

Day 25 – January 25, 2012
"10 mile bike ride=40 minutes. I'm slow! 1,250 yard swim. Today the bike was hard. I felt like my legs were going fast, but I wasn't going anywhere!"

Day 26 – January 26, 2012
"Ran 40 minutes. I had a rough day running today, but I have a long day tomorrow. It's good I saved some energy for that. It's my first group ride!"

Day 27 – January 27, 2012 *"Day off. My arms are sore!"*

Day 28 – January 28, 2012
"Did my 1st group! It was really hard. Almost fell over once, but I caught myself. There was also a strong wind, which made it harder. We rode for 2 hours."

At this point in the training, I could already feel myself changing mentally and physically. My mind became clearer and my physical strength was coming back. When my mind wandered to my past I brought myself back to the present. I was training for a full Ironman just three months sober and without having completed any kind of triathlon. I focused on positive self-talk, continued working on the AA Twelve Steps, and kept training. The Ironman goal wasn't really about the completion or the competition, but rather something that was keeping me sober in that critical first year!

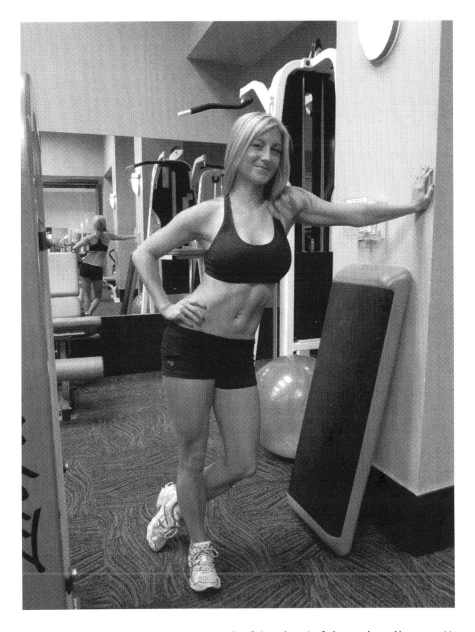

Even though I was training with friends, I felt a loneliness. My training partners weren't recovering alcoholics and the only person who knew my background was my coach and friend. We became extremely close during this time and she became like an older sister to me. We spent everyday together whether swimming, cycling, or running. I was determined to prove to her I wanted to be an athlete and not an alcoholic. She understood my mental struggles and their source. She was able to discern the difference between those struggles and the struggles associated with Ironman training. When I became uncomfortable in a situation, she was able to help me feel better.

My first real challenge was quickly approaching. My coach and I were preparing for a bike tour race in Palm Springs, California. This would be by first cycling race and would be fifty-five miles, which was twenty miles longer than any bike ride I had completed. I was extremely nervous about this race to say the least. I knew I would be slow, but my goal was to simply get through it and finish.

Day 41 – February 10, 2012
"Ran 75 minutes = 8 miles. Longest run so far."

Day 42 – February 11, 2012
"Bike ride, tour de Palm Springs. We were supposed to do 55 miles, but did 45 miles. I got hit by a car, so it delayed our ride. Thankfully it wasn't worse, just some road rash. It really shook me up though. Other than that I felt really good riding. I kept my cadence around 88-90. I look forward to the next long ride."

I didn't let the car clipping incident deter me from continuing the ride. I was determined to finish and my coach was there to help me after I fell. She asked me if I was okay and I told her I was just in shock. She looked me over and told me she thought I could continue which was just what I needed to hear. I had no broken bones, my bike was fine, and so I pushed on. Unless I fainted, puked, or died, I wouldn't stop until I crossed the finish line.

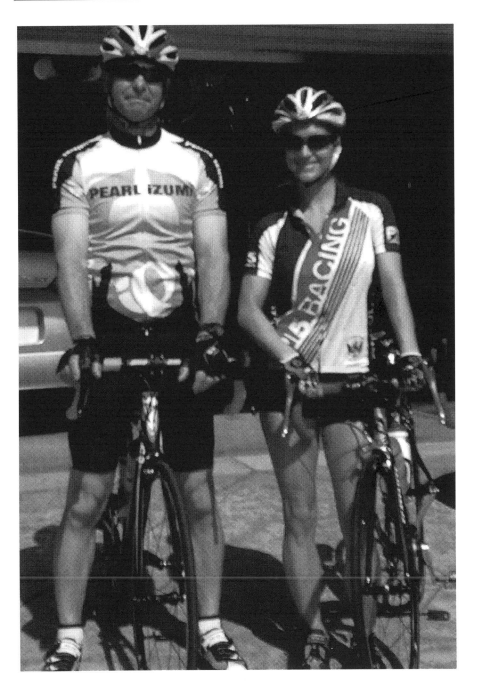

There was something about Ironman training that I never told anyone. The arduous training made me feel proud of myself and that

I was "someone" again which made my confidence return making it easier to be happy about who I was. When I danced I felt strong, confident, and successful. With my new focus in life, I felt the joy and happiness I had before my addiction. I was taking on something very few people accomplish and doing it while recovering from alcoholism. I remembered the euphoria I experienced while performing and decided this would be a new kind of performance where I wouldn't necessarily come out on top. It was the finishing of it that would make me a winner.

My first chance to prove to myself I was mentally and physically stronger was quickly approaching. I was preparing for my very first triathlon and it would be the Olympic distance: 3/4 mile swim, 24 miles on the bike, and a 6.2 mile run.

Day 62 – March 4, 2012
"Race Day, first tri, Desert Tri Olympic Distance. I panicked on the swim, but made it. I felt good on the bike and run though! Swim = 27 minutes, bike = 1 hour 23 minutes, run = 52 minutes. Good times and not an easy course!"

Since this was my first triathlon, my times weren't bad. I was just happy to finish feeling good about the race. The swim proved to be difficult because I wasn't able to breathe with my face in the cold water. I had to backstroke most of the swim but fortunately it was my best stroke at the time. Once I got on the bike I didn't struggle at all and continued to pace myself through the completion of the run. When I crossed the finish line I felt like a true triathlete!

I was beyond proud of myself with my accomplishment, which was something I had not felt in a long time. When I was drinking I never felt any pride and deep down I knew I wasn't on the right course. Now that I had set my first major goal, I gave myself a pat on the back. I learned in sobriety I had to be proud of myself when I worked hard toward a goal. It wasn't an ego trip in any way but a feeling of satisfaction and accomplishment of a job well done. I became a lot stronger after that first triathlon and I began to believe in myself again. I could now visualize myself crossing the finish line of that future Ironman race.

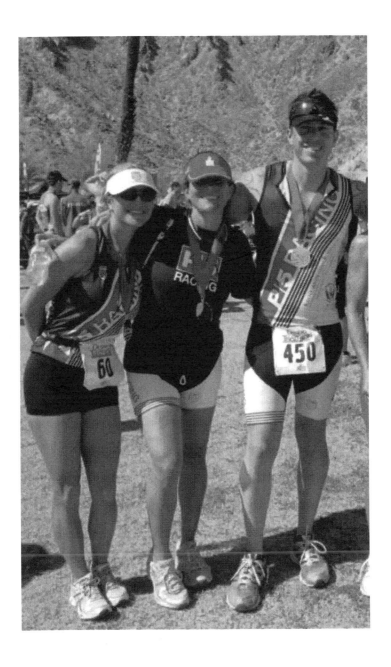

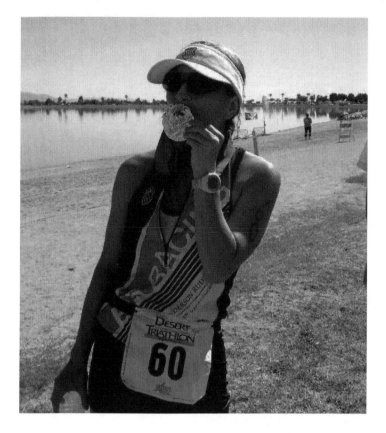

Visualizing the achievement of my goal was important to me because it gave me the motivation, inspiration, and confidence to
make it happen. Many of my training friends talked about the "what
ifs" of the Ironman, which meant they worried about the bad things
that could happen during the long race. I kept telling myself that as
long as I didn't drown, crash on my bike, or break a bone while
running, I was going to finish the race. I learned in AA I shouldn't
future trip about situations. I never thought anything negative about
the future race because I felt doing that would set me up for failure
somewhere along the line. I picture myself winning instead!

March was my most difficult training month. I was about twelve
weeks into training and almost every day consisted of a brick workout. I felt as though I was living on my bike with all the miles I was
logging. I took computrainer classes to improve my cycling. My bike
was set up on a stationary stand and a coach gave me instruction on

pace, cadence, and intensity for ninety minutes. These classes really kicked my butt more than any other part of the training. I dreaded each class knowing how much they were going to hurt, but since it was for the improvement in my cycling, I continued.

Day 82 – March 24, 2012 *"Much needed day off!"*

Day 83 – March 25, 2012
"Accel #4, it was so hard that I got light-headed and stopped before the last two 15 seconds."

Day 84 – March 26, 2012
"Comp 90 minutes, 30 minute run, and masters swim. I sucked at swimming today."

Day 85 - March 27, 2012
"2 hour ride with Raelynn. Did hill repeats, practicing descending.I was still tired afterwards."

Day 86 – March 28, 2012
"Yay, good workout day! 90 minute comp, 20 minute run, and masters swim around 2,700 meters. I felt really good today."

Day 87 – March 29, 2012
"4 hour bike ride, 50 miles! Longest ride I've done so far. I felt really good and could have kept going. I'm really proud of myself."

Day 88 – March 30, 2012
"4,000 meter swim, longest swim I've ever done! I did really good and I feel like I'm getting stronger. BB and spin also."

Day 89 – March 31, 2012
"45 minute run. I did pretty good, just tired."

Day 90 – April 1, 2012
"2 hour run. 13 miles. I did just fine and felt good the whole time."

Day 91 – April 2, 2012
"90 minute comp, 20 minute run, and 2,500 meter masters swim. I suffered in swim. I wanted to give up!"

I had days where I felt amazing and days where I wanted to give up. I had to tell myself over and over that quitting was not an option in this journey. I had never quit anything in my life except drinking and I wasn't about to quit this training. Some days I felt like crying from exhaustion and there were days when my body was so sore I could barely move. But then there were days when everything felt just right and good. This sobriety journey was beginning to test my mental strength. AA taught me it was alright to cry in sobriety because there was no more alcohol to numb the pain. I had never been a big crier, so this seemed strange to me. This is why Ironman training was good for me emotionally.

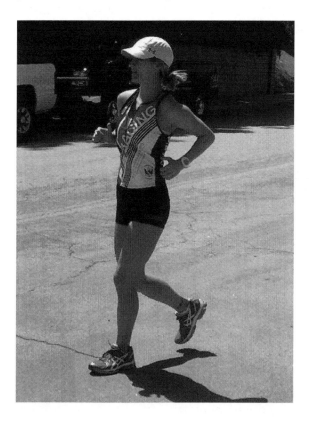

I was out on an eleven mile run with my coach after a long day of cycling, when I suddenly stopped and began crying. My coach asked me what was wrong and I told her I was just so very tired. Since she had been through this type of training, she could empathize with how I was feeling. She suggested I drink, refuel, and take a deep breath. I felt as though I couldn't move my legs at all and all I wanted to do was lie down and go to sleep. The twenty plus hours a week of training made me feel totally depleted. As I drank some water I thought about crossing the finish line and knew then I needed to keep going. I wiped my tears, took a deep breath, and took one step and then another until I had completed the eleven mile run! This epiphany moment made me see I had potential and strength and nothing was going to stop me from training and finishing the Ironman.

After my little breakdown I reached another training milestone in cycling. I completed a seventy mile bike ride!

Day 124 – May 5, 2012
"70 mile bike, 15 minute run. Yay I hit a milestone! I felt fine the whole ride, except for some crotch issues. Can't believe how strong I've become in biking."

There were some issues with sitting on that tiny bike seat for so long. I was completely numb and couldn't imagine what riding 112 miles would feel like. I still felt extremely accomplished and that's all that mattered at the moment. I finally felt like a cyclist, much stronger than when I first started, and could see all the hard work gave me great results.

While putting in the hard training for the Ironman, I still maintained my sobriety and my part-time job as a personal trainer. I trained in the morning and worked with clients after that. There were many moments when I needed to sit down on a stability ball because my legs were so fatigued. I received nothing but support and understanding from my clients on those days. My caloric demand was so high that I had to excuse myself as soon as I felt hunger pangs to refuel my overworked body. My clients were some of my biggest supporters when training got rough.

My training, work, and family and friend relationships were all going well. Unfortunately, my relationship with my boyfriend was not. His addiction was slowly progressing to the point where I couldn't tell if he was drunk or high on drugs. My heart held out hope that he'd make the changes needed to get healthy but my brain pondered breaking up. Everything was going so great in my life and it was hard for me to watch him destroy himself. I was hoping that, like me, he would come out of it before it was too late.

On June 1 I got the phone call I was longing for. My caller ID said it was from my boyfriend and I was expecting to hear that he was drunk or high, but this time it was different. He simply said, "Rochelle, I don't want to do this anymore. I want to get help." I felt as though a huge weight had been lifted off my shoulders and I was flooded with relief. My gut had told me he had a strength within him to beat the addiction. I told him as long as he was serious I would do anything to help him get better. He willingly checked into a rehab program. I was extremely proud of him and looked forward to watching his journey to sobriety. It was at that moment that I knew we were meant to be together forever.

I still had to continue with my Ironman training in spite of my boyfriend's rehab journey. I had to keep focused on my own sobriety journey and self-improvement. I was extremely lucky to have support from my parents and friends on the days when I was really struggling. My parents would remind me of how far I had come and my inner drive to make them proud motivated me to keep moving forward and never look back.

The Ironman race was quickly approaching and was only eight weeks away.

Day 157 – June 7, 2012
"3,000 meter swim and 3 hour bike ride. I wanted to shoot myself on the ride! I was hell. My body is still recovering from Saturday."

Day 158 – June 8, 2012
"60 minute run and 2,500 meter swim. I finally feel like I don't

struggle the whole time during swimming!"

At this time in my training I was starting to question why I was doing what I was doing. The training had intensified and increased to about twenty five hours a week with cycling being my least favorite part. The fatigue was so intense that I was going to bed at 8 o'clock every single night. I was consuming on average 3,000-3,800 calories a day, more on the harder days. My physique was changing, I weighed about 105 pounds at the peak of my training, and carried very low body fat. I looked completely different than when I first became sober.

I had lost all my alcohol bloat and the extra weight I was carrying as a result. My skin began to glow because all of the toxins had left my body. My hair was growing and not thinning like when I was drinking. I recovered from my training activities quicker without alcohol in my system and a healthier diet. My body was in the best shape ever and I finally became completely satisfied with how I looked.

With my Ironman right around the corner, my nerves started to kick in during training. On one particular day I had to do a seventeen mile run, ninety minute bike ride, and a 1,500 meter swim. I was finally at the peak of my training with 100 swimming miles, 2,675 cycling miles, and 470 running miles! These statistics helped put in perspective all the hard work I had put in. With only four weeks to go until race day, I was more confident than ever.

A Century Ride is a bike ride of 100 miles or more within twelve hours. I completed my third such ride on July 4th and could finally visualize myself completing the 112 mile cycling section of the Ironman. From my first ride where I couldn't even switch gears to completing three rides of 100 miles gave me a great confidence boost. I continued to stay focused and motivated while counting the days until the big race.

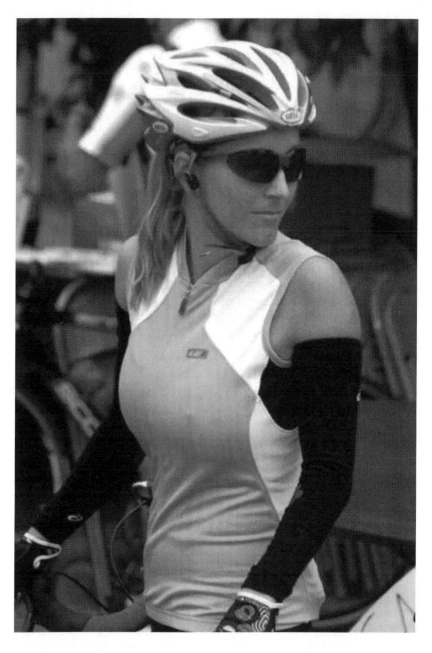

I finally reached a point in my sobriety when I felt comfortable telling my story to the public. Our local newspaper, The Ventura County Star, loved my story so much that they decided to write a full article about it. What a thrill to see my face on the front page and an entire section dedicated to my story of recovery and training for an Ironman. Being a recovering alcoholic is something very personal and not something a lot of people want to admit to, but I wanted to help others as I made my journey to sobriety. One individual was so moved by the article that he sent me a private Facebook message telling me how my story had helped him. I knew at that time I needed to continue on my journey and follow through on my commitment to complete that Ironman triathlon. I hoped the article would be the first of many.

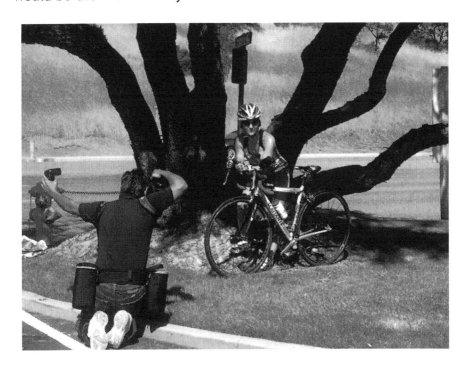

Early in the morning, on July 15th, I was driving to visit my boyfriend in rehab which was about a ninety minute drive. I supported him in his recovery by going every Sunday during visiting hours. During the drive I changed lanes at the same time as another car, we crashed into each other, and I lost complete control of my car. All I remember is that I saw the center divider coming my way, my head hit my side window frame, and then nothing. When I regained consciousness my foot was stuck under the brake pedal and my first thoughts were hoping no bones were broken thus preventing me from competing in the Ironman. My car was totaled, my foot was bruised, and there was blood running down my leg from the shattered glass. Other than that I was safe, hadn't been drinking and driving, so would get through this accident and move forward toward my big goal.

I went to the doctor to get my injuries evaluated and thankfully I had no broken bones. My doctor told me that I sustained less injuries due to my physical training. He gave me the green light to continue training and go to the race. I felt like someone was looking out for me that day and that I could continue on toward my Ironman goal.

On July 26th, I headed out to Sonoma, California, for my big race. I had butterflies in my stomach the entire drive there. All I could think about were my nerves and becoming an Ironman.

> Day 207 – July 27, 2012
> *"40 minute bike ride, 20 minute run, then swam 20 minutes in the river. I feel much more comfortable now. I'm more than ready for tomorrow and God will let me have a smooth, fun race.*
> *1) Have fun!*
> *2) Eat and hydrate*
> *3) Pace myself*
> *4) Think positive*
> *5) Dig deep and be strong! Look how far I've come!"*

The day before the race I wrote down five things to remember while racing. I was an optimist, so I was already visualizing myself crossing the finish line. There was no doubt in my mind I wouldn't finish and had no plans to give up even if my body screamed to stop. Tomorrow would be my day to own it and prove to everyone how far I had come in only ten months. I had heard stories of how the Ironman changed people's lives, but wasn't ready for the change it would give me.

My alarm went off at 4:00 a.m. on the morning of July 28, with visions of becoming an Ironman going through my head. My big day had arrived at last! I grabbed all of my gear, headed out the door, and headed to the transition area to set up and fuel for the race.

With that done, I had an hour to spare, and only felt excitement about what the path before me. I was prepared and confident I would finish. I just wanted to get started.

I zipped up my wetsuit and put on my swim cap. My parents, who had come along to support me, were taking tons of pictures. My brother surprised me by showing up the night before after telling me he couldn't come. My aunt and godson came to see me finish. My boyfriend was still in rehab so was unable to join us. I would have loved to have him there but he needed to stay in his program and get well. I would miss his presence but my already large support crew would help me through this grueling competition. I was ready to show them what I was made of.

I heard the announcer call us to the start of the swim and my heart began to pound with ferocity. I took a deep breath, told myself that I was more than ready, reminded myself how far I had come, and was ready to go for it. I was so nervous that when the gun went off, I urinated right in my wetsuit. My excitement and nerves were overwhelming.

I ran to the water's edge, dove in, and took the first stroke into my Ironman race day journey. With every stroke and breath, I took in the beautiful scenery around me. I stayed relaxed during the swim, got into my pace quickly, and tried to avoid getting hit or kicked in the face. The swim course was two 1.2 mile loops with parts that were so shallow that I had to stand up. On my second lap I could see the finish line about 300 meters ahead of me and I was ecstatic to have made it through. I came out of the water in one hour and 21 minutes, nine minutes faster than I had expected.

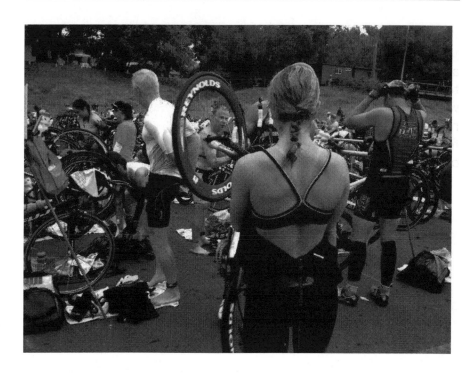

Since I wasn't going against the clock, I took a long time to transition into the bike event. I wanted to make sure I was one hundred percent prepared for this portion of the race. I hopped on my bike, clipped in, and was ready to conquer the 112 miles ahead of me. At mile thirty, my back began hurting and I realized I was going to have to tough it out to the end. The heat was almost unbearable, about 90°, which caused nausea and fatigue to set in. I drank liquids every thirty minutes and refueled every forty five. I had to stay focused on hydration and fuel for the remainder of the race or I would be in serious trouble.

With the added hydration, I had to stop at every single bathroom during the 112 miles. At mile seventy I knew I still had a long way to go. My brain was turning to mush and I couldn't think straight and everything on my body hurt, but I kept pedaling. I would persevere no matter what. I talked to myself during the ride to keep my sanity. I knew I was struggling but remembered how far I had come to get to this point. I felt as though I was in a dream and my dream was becoming a reality with every mile that passed.

With two miles to go and a sudden rush, I felt like a million bucks. I just wanted to get off that bike and run! The run was my safety net and favorite part of the event. I hit my brakes, unclipped, and ran to the next transition area. I was so tired I couldn't remember where I set up my gear. It took me ten minutes just to find my running shoes, I threw down my bike and vowed I wouldn't ride it for a year! I laced up my shoes and took off running. I was ready to own those 26.2 miles and enjoy every moment of it.

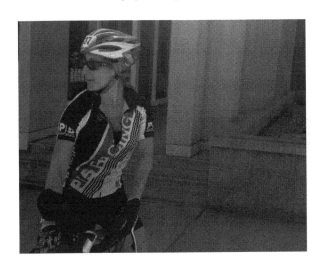

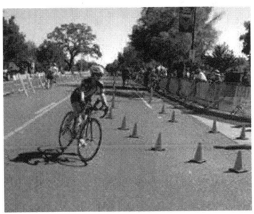

During Ironman competition, electronic music devices aren't allowed so as I ran I listened to the cheering spectators and the pounding of my feet. I breathed evenly in order to relax and enjoy this portion of the race. I refueled every thirty minutes and continued hydrating often. The temperatures were starting to cool down so I started to feel good again. I kept my pace during the three loop course and enjoyed seeing my cheering squad each time I came around. Their support and encouraging words kept me motivated to keep going and push harder.

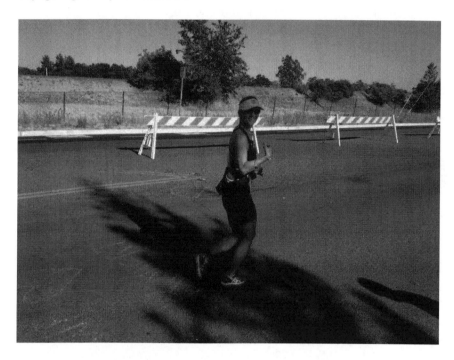

I set out to enjoy that portion of the race and enjoy it I did. I never struggled because I stuck to my planned pace and stayed steady and relaxed. When I reached 13.1 miles I told myself I was halfway through the run and to keep going. I pictured my parents' proud faces watching me cross that final finish line. I thought about those back home, tracking my progress electronically. At one point in the run there was nobody around me. I looked around, realized I had only two miles to go and got a huge smile on my face. I thought to myself, "I freaking did it, I'm winning my life back."

As I neared the finish line of my third running loop and the conclusion of my first Ironman, I could hear the cheer of the spectators. I looked ahead and could see the finish line about fifty feet away.

With tears streaming down my face, enjoying the last few moments, taking it all in, I took my last stride and crossed the finish line of my first Ironman triathlon. I raised my hands in triumph and said to myself, "Rochelle, you are an Ironman."

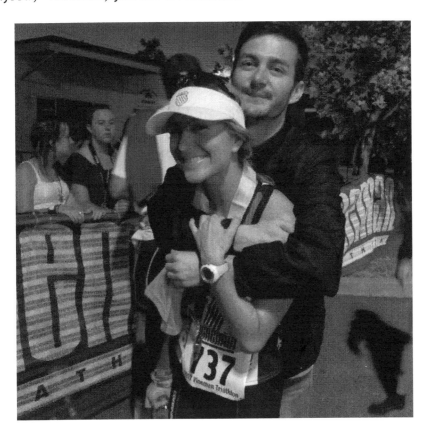

There are very few words to describe how I felt at that defining moment. I hadn't won an Ironman competition but had won my life back. Crossing the finish line was not only the best moment of my life, but more importantly, it saved my life. I was truly an athlete again and a sober one at that. Ironman, without a doubt, had left an indelible mark on my soul and life.

That mark would carry me onto newer and better things. I felt like I could conquer anything that was set before me. The support of my family, boyfriend, and friends would further bolster those feelings. Without the guidance of my coach and mentor, the journey might have ended up differently. She was there for me through my addiction and then through my sobriety journey to becoming a true athlete and Ironman. I had regained my self-confidence, physical and mental strength, and new focus in life. Ironman, you forever changed me, saved my life and for that I am grateful. I am a sober Ironman.

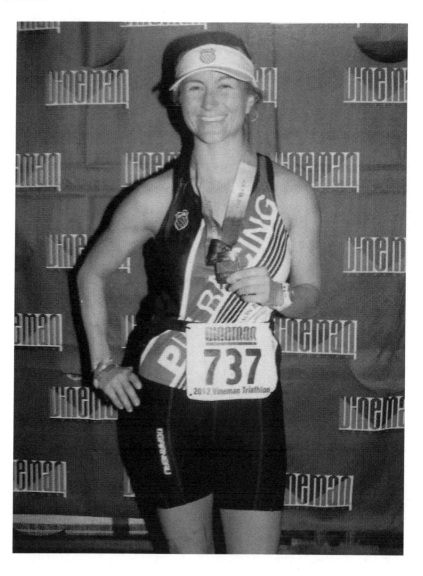

Chapter 7
Life after Ironman and the Road Ahead

After the epic finish of my first Ironman triathlon, many people have asked if I was finished competing. Since I had done many other race distances on top of the big one people assumed there was nothing more to achieve. I decided that for me, there is no real finish line. The Ironman was only the beginning of a new life for me. After Ironman I set some new life goals, some of which were fitness related and others for my life in general. I wanted people to be inspired and motivated by both my story and daily goals.

I had found a new passion in life, one of fitness and triathlons. Fitness has become more than just an activity or type of exercise I enjoy doing. It is at the core of who I am. I live and breathe fitness on a daily basis. I live to help and inspire others through my story and personal training.

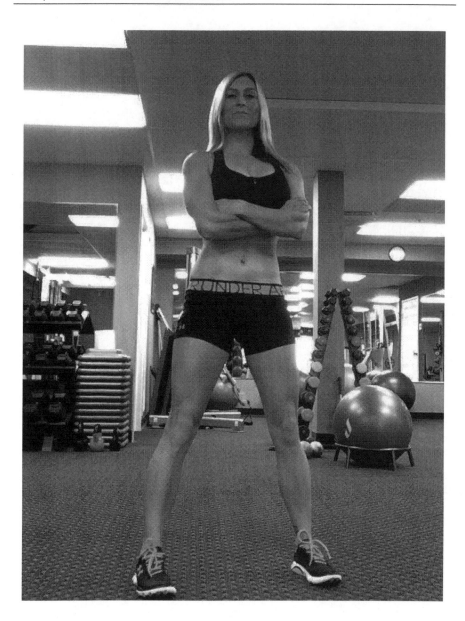

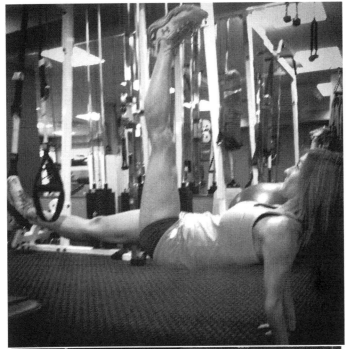

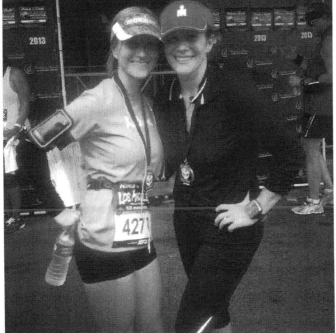

My life was continuing in the right direction but I had no idea that there were more great things to come. I entered an all-women's Under Armour competition in the hopes of becoming a finalist. Contestants were required to set a goal and post videos and pictures of the achievement. The competition lasted eight weeks and I gave it my all. I chose a thirty day running streak for the first four weeks and a cycling challenge for the next four. I wanted to stand out to the judging team in order to become a finalist for the grand prize.

After eight weeks of working hard, I was more than thrilled to discover that I had become one of ten finalists in the competition. I was proud that I had set out with a goal and was able to accomplish it. I didn't win the grand prize, but I became an Under Armour ambassador which came as a total surprise to me. I would be able to represent their brand and motivate others.

Another major goal had been to be a trainer on the hit television show, "The Biggest Loser." The show is a combination of my three passions: fitness, helping others, and my love for being in front of the camera. One of my role models, Dolvett Quince, was a trainer on the show. He trained and helped many people lose weight. I started following him on   social media, making comments, and liking his posted pictures. I was excited when he began following be back. I dreamed of meeting him one day. I learned that he was going to be doing a book signing near me so I went early to be the first person in line. When he saw me he immediately recognized me, greeted me by name, and asked how my sobriety and training had been going. It was an amazing moment for me to meet a fitness mentor.

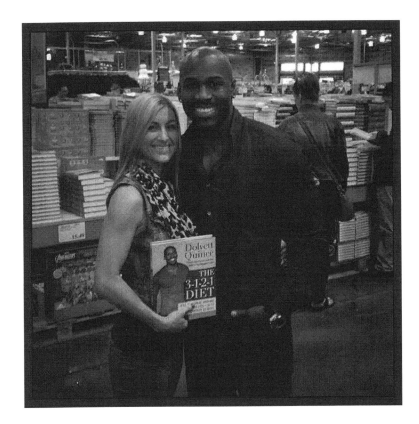

After my Ironman I really wanted to continue in my fitness excellence and set some new goals. In 2013, I ran my sixth marathon in Los Angeles and set a personal record. The long training began to wear on me and fatigue and boredom made me want to try something different. I decided to try sprint distance races.

I began my sprint distance journey in November of 2013. I ran my first official 5K on Thanksgiving morning, coming in at 23:42, averaging 7:37 pace and placing 7th in my age group. I was very surprised at being able to go under an eight-minute mile. I was instantly hooked and gained a new confidence in my running ability. My new goal for 2014 was to place as many times as possible and one day get on the podium in 1st-3rd place.

During 2014, I gave every ounce of energy I had into training for sprint distance. I ran my first 5K in January and came in first place in my age group at 22:46. The first place for that race brought back memories from when I won dance competitions and I could feel my competitive side finally returning. I wanted to keep the ball rolling so continued running and triathlon training.

I placed first in my age in another 5K so I felt ready to try the sprint distance for a triathlon which consists of a 750 meter swim, 20K bike ride, and 5K run. My goal was to place in the top three and get on the podium. I swam so hard that I was completely out of breath as I transitioned to the bike portion of the race. I knew I would have to really dig deep, push as hard as possible, and get to the run which was my strongest event. I transitioned to the run, took off, felt strong, and was having the time of my life.

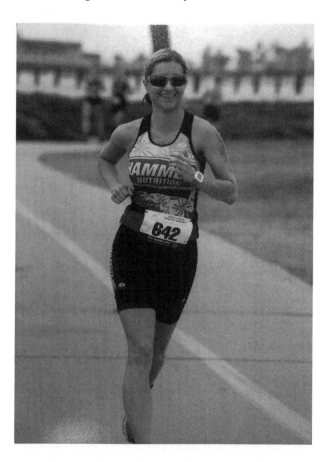

When I was about 200 meters from the finish line, I spotted a girl from my age group just ahead. I knew I had to really pick up the pace in order to catch her before the finish line. I increased my pace to a 6:30 mile pace, gritted my teeth and held on to pass her with 1/10th of a mile to go. After I finished I learned that by passing her I went from fourth to third place. I had made the podium on my first sprint triathlon!

I kept competing in sprint triathlons and placed in twelve races throughout 2014. I never imagined that I would be competing because I had never thought of myself as a natural born athlete. I had a great work ethic and that was the key to my success. I trained hard and visualized winning races. I always tell my clients that if they can envision achieving a goal then they will be able to do it.

I still had the desire to get my story out to others so that they could be inspired and motivated. A client mentioned a contest through Women's Running Magazine where an inspirational story was submitted and the winner would be on the cover of one publication. There were over 2,000 entries and I was chosen as one of ten finalists. The final winner was chosen based on social media voting. I received a lot of support and votes, but it wasn't enough to be chosen for first place. I was a little disappointed but didn't worry because I was sure that there would be other opportunities to get my story to the public. I continued my usual positive attitude and didn't give up on my dream. It just wasn't my time to grace the cover of a magazine.

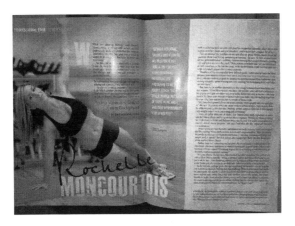

A wise friend once told me that someday a great opportunity would come knocking at my door and he was spot on! At the end of 2014 I was contacted by Shape Magazine to do an article about my story for their website. I was literally jumping up and down with excitement. Shape Magazine was my favorite magazine at that time and I was going to be a part of it. When the story came out online, I got many positive responses. People began finding me on Instagram and Facebook social media to tell me how my story was both helpful and inspirational. These responses brought tears to my eyes because I was finally helping others with their addiction troubles and giving them hope.

With the positive responses from the online article, I began to think about other ways to get my story out to a wider audience. After much thought I decided that another goal was to write a complete and detailed book about my addiction and recovery story. Since I had never written a book this journey would definitely take me into new territory!

While in the process of writing my book, I had some amazing moments in my life because of sobriety. I was able to land a job with a brand new fitness company called Aaptiv. Aaptiv is an App that allows someone to train with a trainer anywhere at anytime. I instantly fell in love with the idea and have watched the company grow. I feel in my element at the recording studio, recording fitness classes for members to listen and workout too! I love being able to help people achieve their goals and dreams.

While maintaining my personal training job and a coach on Aaptiv, I also came across a few more major milestones. I got married to the man of my dreams on May 21, 2016. It was without a doubt one of the best days of my life. My husband and I were also blessed and surprised with the gift of twin girls. Never in my life did I expect to have twins(since they don't run in the family). I went through my pregnancy staying active up until week thirty. My waist went from 25 inches to 45! I also had a rough recovery from my C-section, but it was worth every moment. We welcomed two beautiful baby girls into the world on January 25, 2017. My husband and I fell in love instantly with Maci Jolie and Morgan Jane. I now have the family I always wanted because of my sobriety.

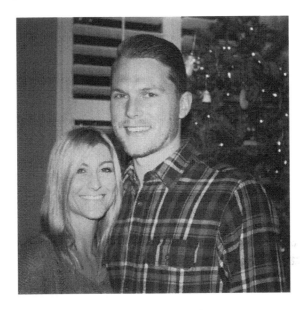

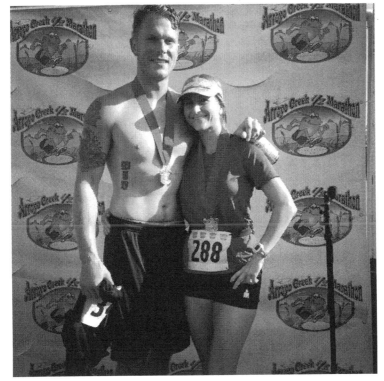

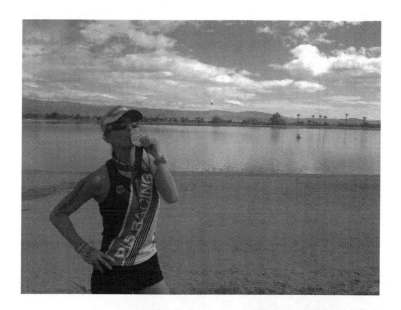

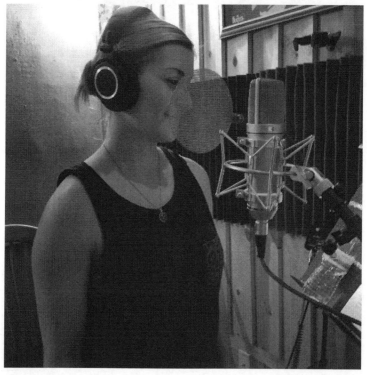

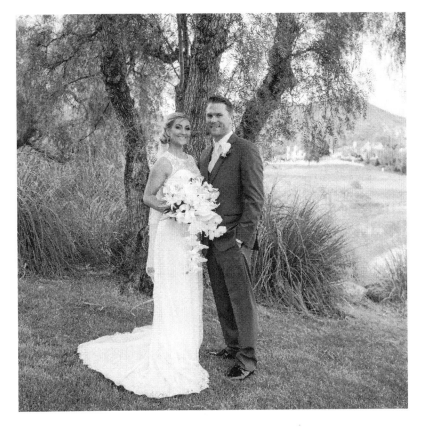

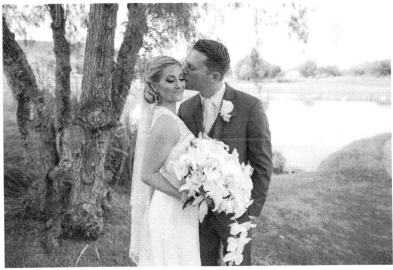

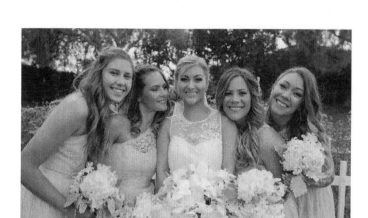

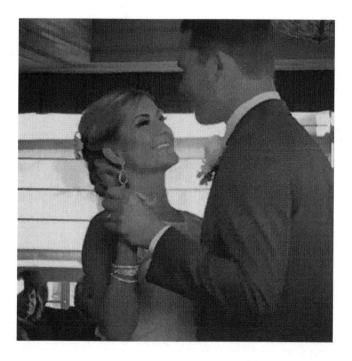

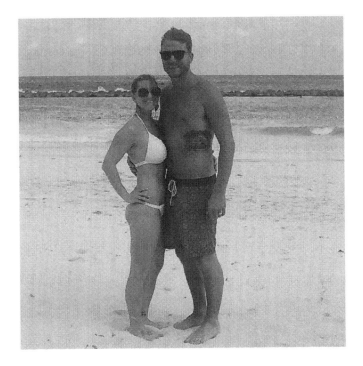

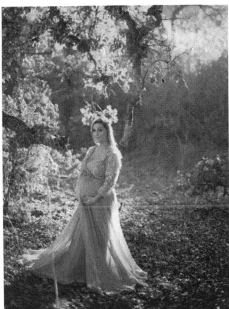

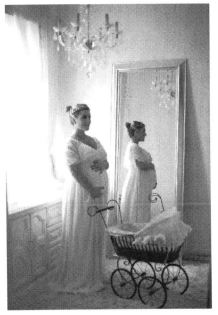

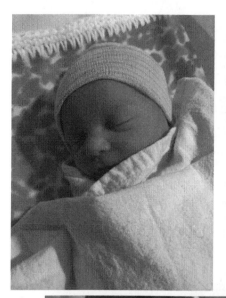
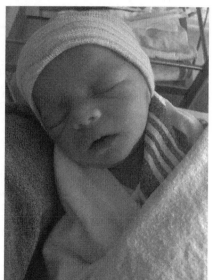
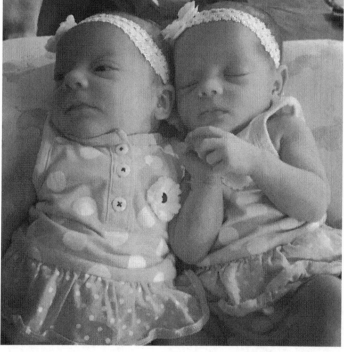

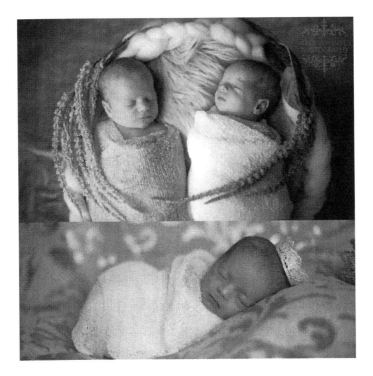

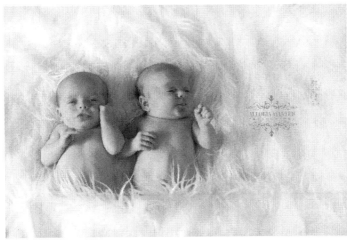

My main purpose in writing this book was to inspire and motivate others who may be going through an addiction or some other kind of struggle. I want them to know with the proper help and hard work, recovery is possible. This book would be an avenue of hope for those who may feel hopeless and a tool to help find courage to dig deep in order to save a life. I made the necessary changes and now I am living a life I only dreamed about.

Readers of my book would be encouraged to think about how bad they want something and then to go after it. Readers would be able to use their struggle as motivation to push harder to achieve what they want out of life. My book would encourage readers to get the necessary help they need immediately so as to defeat those addiction demons. I want them to take charge of their lives and make it amazing. I went from a talented dancer, to a drunk girl at a club, to an Ironman triathlete. I went from the bottom of life's worse pit to the healthy, happy, balanced person I am today and others will be able to learn from my journey.

I would also like to build and create a triathlon clothing line that combines fashion and comfort. All of these goals were made possible because of sobriety and finding a passion during Ironman. It was all because I wanted to change and make my dreams come true. Through hard work, determination, courage, and commitment, you can too.

I am Alcoholic to Ironman.

Made in the USA
San Bernardino, CA
21 February 2018